Lewy Body Dementia

Survival

and Me

Author: KEVIN QUAID

Lewy Body Dementia Patient

By Kevin Quaid

0035386-1526041

Email: kevinquaid9@gmail.com

ISBN-13;978-1720495758

ISBN-10;1720495750

Copyright© Kevin Quaid 2018

Edited by Noreen Quaid, Australia.

Printed by Kanturk Printers, Kanturk, Co. Cork. Ireland.

ID 8554431

I

am not

a victim of

Lewy Body Dementia

I am

a

<u>SURVIVOR</u>

TABLE OF CONTENTS

Lewy Body Dementia, Survival *and* Me

Dedication

This book is dedicated to my very special cousin Theresa Quaid Myers, without whose constant encouragement and support this book may never have been written. I am so grateful to her for sharing her inspiration and courage with me.

Theresa became an angel the day this book was ready to be published.

Best Wishes

14/6/2024

ACKNOWLEDGEMENTS

This journey was one that I could not have taken on my own without the love and encouragement shown to me by family and friends.

Chapter 18 was written by my wonderful children and stepchildren, Noreen, Pat, Kevin, Declan, Shane and Michelle, my fantastic brother Tom and my true friend Mike. I cried a lot reading it as your love for me is so real.

My beautiful daughter Noreen for editing the book.

My good friend Jimmy for his brilliant help and support, not just now but always.

My beautiful Grandchildren, Hollie, Charlie, Liam, Victoria and any others who may come along.

I would especially like to thank Dr Dennise Broderick for her invaluable enthusiastic encouragement from the beginning.

Helena, my beautiful wife who is at my side through it all, good and bad and whose constant love and support is simply amazing.

I also wish to thank most sincerely the following people who have helped me along this journey with Lewy Body Dementia.

Dr. Donal O'Riordan GP

Staff at Egmont Medical Centre

Dr. Orna O'Toole Consultant Neurologist

Dr James Kinahan Consultant Psychiatrist

PJ O'Neill Counsellor

The Crystal Project

Care Bright Centre

Foreword

Lewy Body Dementia (LBD) is a disease of the mind and body that robs the sufferer of all the "joie de vivre" this world has to offer. Due to the very nature of LBD the journey to diagnosis alone can be fraught with frustrations and anger as sufferers seeking answers are often met with obstacles or misdiagnoses. Final diagnosis may in fact only come after years of symptomatic presentation.

This book provides a personal account of one man's journey through LBD diagnosis and how he lives daily with this disease. It is an honest and authentic narrative of what LBD does to the life of an otherwise vibrant and active person. In his own words,

Kevin portrays to all who will read this book, the reality of Lewy Body Dementia. He describes the changes that take place in both the mind and the body as this illness ravages his life one day at a time.

But this is also a book of hope, a book with the very word "survival" in the title. Hope is a gift for anyone suffering a degenerative and progressive illness. Kevin provides this hope through recounting his experiences as a man with LBD, experiences that will give identification to those fellow sufferers upon reading this book. Hope comes for most when we do not feel alone and identification bonds us in togetherness. This book is an exercise in togetherness for all who will read it and share Kevin's life through his own lens.

Hope is also necessary for the families, friends and loved ones of all suffering with LBD. This book will give hope to them through the words of Kevin's wife (his now carer) and the words of many loved ones who have contributed. I am one such person, having known Kevin for many years as Goddaughter and niece to his wife.

Lewy Body Dementia is progressive. Lewy Body Dementia is degenerative. Lewy Body Dementia has no cure. Kevin takes the reality of this illness and lays it bare for all to read in the pages of this book. He authentically and courageously shares with us his journey with LBD desiring that this book will help others to find hope in a situation that may otherwise seem hopeless.

Dr. Dennise Broderick.

Chapter One

A little boy from a small village

As I start to write this book I am 54 years old, born in a small village in County Limerick in Ireland in 1963. I am the eldest of six children - five boys and one girl. My parents were both hardworking people, my mother looked after the family and a small local shop in the village, and my father ran a small building company. That time there was more of an interest in the quality of the job than any finish line.

This book *LEWY BODY DEMENTIA, SURVIVAL and ME* is an idea I wanted to make a reality following on from my diagnosis in May 2017 at the age of 53 when my Neurologist sent me for a DaTscan and confirmed the presence of Lewy Bodies in my brain.

The opinions and thoughts are my own unless otherwise stated and are in no way meant to hurt, frighten or alarm people but simply to try and make sense of this terrible disease.

My new reality came after years of different diagnoses, some of which I now know were misdiagnosed and some of which have led up to where I am today. At the time of diagnosis with LBD (that's short for Lewy Body Dementia) I had at that time been diagnosed with Parkinson's Disease for about two years, but more about that in a later chapter. Diagnosed so young with LBD and at such an early stage may give you an insight into what to expect, because a lot of people do not get diagnosed until it's too late.

In fact, in a lot of cases, it is only after death when an autopsy is performed that LBD is confirmed. That is just a brief note on the dementia side and one that I will go into in greater detail in section three of the book.

Suicide is not a selfish act

Some people may not agree with the above statement and others will, but as I have already said this is my thinking on it and I am going to be honest and true to myself as I write this book. The reason for the section on survival is because of my own fights with suicide, and also the amount of lives it takes and destroys. One thing I really hate is that some people believe and say that suicide is a very selfish act. In my opinion SUICIDE IS NOT A SELFISH ACT, but more about this in later chapters.

The reason I have this belief may not make sense to you without going into my complete life story. I want to touch on a lot of the things that happened in my life, some good, some bad and in some cases very bad, staying in my mind up to this present day, and I often wonder have they shaped the way my mind is today?

The biggest question of all, is how and why did I get Lewy Body Dementia?

1. Was I born with it?
2. Is it hereditary?
3. Was it the result of how I lived my life?
4. Was it because of what happened to me?
5. Was it just hard luck?
6. Or was it the path already mapped out for my journey through this life

Hopefully I will get to answer some of these questions, probably not all but at least some. I suppose the first thing that I will try to do is fill you in on how my mind developed from as far back as I can remember.

I had a happy childhood and as I said my parents worked hard, we were never short of anything, but nothing was ever wasted either. At Christmas, Easter and Birthdays we were always made to feel very special and every year my parents ensured we went on a family holiday.

I was particularly close to my Grandparents and wound up calling my Grandfather 'GAG' (short for Gaggand because as a child I found it difficult to pronounce Grandad). The first time I remember thinking that this world was cruel was a couple of days after starting school. I already hated the school and could not figure out why a happy child would be put into such a terrible place.

We were out playing in the grass at break time when who should I see walking across the road only my Gag. Oh, how my heart filled with happiness and joy, the thought even struck me, was he going to rescue me from this terrible place? But no…. he waved and smiled but kept on walking, so I had nothing better to do but wave back at him with a tear in my eye…. I said to all the young scholars who were out playing with me.... *look everyone.... that's 'GAG'.... there's 'GAG'.* To my horror they all started laughing and mocking me and one of them called me Professor Gaggands.

Right there and then my world fell apart and I felt so alone for the first time in my life. Of course, this nickname 'Gags' stuck with me throughout school and to this day I still hate it. School and home life continued pretty normal. I hated lessons but did OK in school and went on to finish my Leaving Certificate . I had some good friends and got on pretty well with my teachers, so it wasn't all bad.

Dad built a new house and we moved just a few miles over the road from the rented shop. I was so excited by the move and felt very happy about it, living in a beautiful place but I was harbouring a very dark and as I thought at the time a very shameful secret. I had been sexually abused, not by any relative but someone everyone knew. Let's face it.... we lived in a small parish and it's not that everyone knew that he was a sexual predator but that everyone knew everyone. I didn't tell anyone, because just imagining the hurt to his family and the scandal of it all just filled me with fear and dread and anyway who would believe me! I knew I would never pluck up the courage to tell even though I could give a very graphic description of what had happened. For a child, this secret was a very heavy burden to carry and live with each and every day. I can say that it was the first time in my life that I thought about suicide, because of the guilt and shame in my head and remember I was only a child.

Growing up, even from a very young age it wasn't uncommon for me to faint if I was hurt or if I heard any talk of someone else being hurt or in an accident. One of my earliest memories of being very sick was when I was in National school and was possibly in third class. I along with some others in my class had to go to hospital in Limerick to have some teeth removed. Something happened there, and I wonder could it have affected me later on in life.

I remember that day very clearly and was very nervous as I sat in the waiting room that morning, with my Dad and Mam and just wanted to get the whole horrible episode over with as quickly as possible. I knew once I was put to sleep I wouldn't feel nervous anymore.

When it came to my turn to go into the dentist, I was glad in a way thinking, it will not be long now until I am put to sleep, but when I went in, they said I would have to wait a few minutes as they had to change the gas because it had run out. They eventually put the gas mask on me and to this day I can remember inhaling the gas for what seemed like forever and ever…. I was eagerly waiting to fall asleep…but alas for me no sleep! Then someone left the room to change the gas again, as they felt it wasn't working and I certainly knew it wasn't. I was eventually put to sleep; my teeth were removed, and I was taken into recovery. I learned later that they could not wake me up, my school buddies who were called into the dentist after me had all woken up and were going home but I was still asleep.

They were eventually successful in waking me however, I was very drowsy but allowed to go home. I was waking and sleeping for hours and even though I was still drowsy I was allowed to get up around 7 o'clock that evening. Within minutes I got violently sick, vomiting up a large pan of blood and of course the Doctor was called, arriving without delay he gave my Dad and Mam instructions on how best to deal with me - a very sick little boy that night. The Doctor had made enquires to the hospital with regards to my severe reaction. This procedure was undertaken on a regular basis in that hospital with little or no adverse effects. He found that the wrong gas had been used on me, but it had not been used on any of the other children attending the hospital that day.

Did that have an effect on my brain?

Chapter Two
Loneliness is a personal thing

Sometimes, even if I am surrounded by family and friends I still can feel incredibly alone.

The year before I did my Leaving Certificate in the early 1980s , my Dad got me a summer job in a hardware shop about 25 miles from home. I got on very well there and they must have been pleased with my performance because when I left to go back to school in September, the boss then told me to come back the day I finish my Leaving Cert. How fantastic and not only that but I also had my first car, a Mini Clubman so in lots of ways I felt very lucky indeed.

The car belonged to a girl from Australia called Mary who had come on holidays a couple of times but eventually ended up extending a trip and she came to live with us for 6 months. The entire family fell in love with Mary as did I, she worked as an Air Hostess and not only a beautiful person on the inside but also drop dead gorgeous. The day that Mary left to go back home to Australia is another day that I will never forget. It was heart- breaking. She was going back to the other side of the world and I can honestly say that for me it was like a death in the family. You know what I mean, it was that pure raw feeling of loss in the pit of your stomach. I felt lonely and grieved for months after Mary and I am thrilled to tell you that she is still a lifelong friend and we meet and chat pretty often.

Loneliness is a very personal thing and when you combine loneliness and grief with a deep-seated hatred about yourself, it can and is a very lonely and dangerous place to be. Not too unlike some days I have now living with LBD. In fact, the feelings are very similar, so right here and now I can connect the feelings of being alone today and being alone as a child.

Anyway, back to my new job and my car, free from school, money in my pocket therefore what could go wrong as all was right with my world – but had I spoken too soon.

Another lad started in the company around the same time as I did. Within my first couple of days it became obvious that I was picking up things faster than he was, especially on the computers. He was not happy, was a lot stronger than me, quite cunning and it didn't take long for me to realise he was a bully. On a regular basis, we would have to tidy the store or do some other work out of sight of both our customers and fellow staff, that's when it began. He started to play this game where we would hit one another in the shoulder to see who was the strongest. I didn't want to look weak, so I went along with it for as long as I could manage thinking it would pass but unfortunately this went on for weeks and many is the day I ended up in the toilets crying with the pain from the beating that he gave me. He said that if I told anyone, he and his brothers would kill me and the best thing for me to do was leave.

Once again, I felt I could tell no one as my Dad helped me secure this fine job and also I had been telling everyone how much I loved it. The only thing left to do was try to avoid him as much as possible which was not easy in this working environment. The beatings continued, not every day but at least every second day until it got so bad that I could hardly lift my left arm.

I was only 17 years old and in a desperate state when the thought of suicide entered my head for a second time. At that time, it seemed to me the only way out, but as luck would have it, a couple of staff members noticed that things with me were not quite right. I later learned that they had been secretly keeping an eye on me, watching and listening to my behaviour whilst at work. Eventually they took me aside and asked me what was wrong, even though I was half afraid to tell them anything at first, they persevered, and I finally blurted everything out. My boxing partner was spoken to quietly.... I THINK! The beatings stopped from then on and within a month, my man had left the company.

Happy days, the world for me was a wonderful place again. I got on well in the job and was keen to learn. It wasn't long before I was filling orders and doing small quotations on my own and I also had a good rapport with the customers. I moved out of home even though my parents discouraged it, but looking back now it was the right thing to do. I was staying out late, doing my own thing and they were probably worrying a lot about me.

Time and life rolled on and I moved from place to place, one job better than the next but never staying for long in any job, four years was the longest time I spent in any of them as I think I got bored easily. I drank quite heavily during my late teens and early twenties, it blocked out a lot of the hurt and guilt and when I was drunk I believed I had found my happy place.

My first ever stay in hospital was in the early eighties when I had to have a knee operation for a sports injury resulting in damaged cartilage. That time there was no keyhole surgery available and both sides of my knee had to be cut open. I ended up with a total of

24 stitches and was in a full cast from my groin to my ankle for six weeks. I was a smoker in those days and imagine smoking was allowed in the hospital ward at that time, hard to believe!

I decided to move to England in the middle of the 1980s, for better weather as they say (only joking) and I travelled with Slatterys', as they ran a bus service at that time from Tralee to London.

I remember the day I arrived in Victoria Road in London. I had travelled by myself, all but penniless and knew nobody but I had made arrangements through a friend of a friend that I would be met off of Slatterys' Bus. True to his word, a very nice man met me off the bus and took me to the tube station to go to North London to a place called Deptford, but My God, when I say the tube station......I thought I had landed on Mars. We arrived at the said destination and I booked into the Bed & Breakfast next to what they called a Dosshouse, so you can imagine the condition of the B & B, let's just say it wasn't like I was staying at The Ritz.

Once again, I found myself alone, only this time in a different country, sharing a room in a bed & breakfast with 6 complete strangers. As I lay there in these new surroundings, I was beginning to wonder if I had made the right decision. For the first time in my life, I missed my family but felt that I couldn't even call them as all of this was of my own making and our relationship had become somewhat strained at this point, but when you are at rock bottom, the only way is up. The following morning I dusted myself off and first things first I went looking for a job, this was actually no bother to me as I had luckily always been successful in securing employment. Within a matter of a day or two I got a job, got settled into a nice flat and started to enjoy life once again.

I made some new and I have to say very good friends, got married, moved back to Ireland and had 3 wonderful children, Noreen, Pat and Kevin. Life rolled on, the years passed by and the marriage ended. During this time of my life a lot of things seemed to be getting out of control and as the years went by I seemed to be getting deeper and deeper into debt even though I was actually never out of work. Struggling trying to get out of debt and putting my life back on track was tough, it was like being in the middle of a whirlwind that I couldn't find my way out of. I eventually joined a 12-step programme to try and bring some order back into my life, which it did and I am very grateful for.

I was now a Dad who was separated and picking up my 3 beautiful children every Friday evening was the highlight of my week. We always did something as a family or went somewhere fun. Dropping them off on Sunday evenings led to tears both for me and the children and I would eagerly look forward to the next weekend and remember this was a time with no mobile phones, so no texts or Facebook to keep tabs on one another during the week like you can now.

I went to America on holiday in the early 1990s, for 2 weeks to my Uncle Dave, his lovely wife Olive and family. I had such a good time there, made all the more exciting because of the fact that I had always adored my Uncle Dave. While there I saw an opportunity to maybe get some work, make some good money and finally get out of debt. I came back home, sorted out what I needed to sort out and headed off to my well-paid job in Chicago.

I didn't stay there very long as I missed my children so much and was lonely and homesick. I had earned a little cash and had saved enough so that when I returned home I started up a small but successful concrete business.

I was beginning to settle down, living in a lovely place and had 3 beautiful children but I found myself troubled by the memories of the sexual abuse of my past. I was advised that counselling might help, and I started to visit a brilliant therapist called PJ O'Neill in Tralee County Kerry, who I found to be absolutely excellent and he helped me deal with and work through these issues.

With his help I actually met and confronted the person who abused me, and this gave me the chance to prove to myself and my inner child that I had done nothing wrong and in fact this other person was completely responsible. I was able to forgive this person but most important of all was that I was able to forgive myself.

This of course didn't happen overnight, but it eventually did, showing me how not to be a victim therefore it pretty much set me free.

Around this time, late 1990s, I met and married the love of my life whose support is

invaluable. Since then I have always said &
hold dear the following prayer –

God grant me the serenity,
To accept the things, I cannot change.
Courage to change the things I can and
The wisdom to know the difference.

Chapter Three
Did it all start in Jersey?

Everyone you know will in some way shape or
form be fighting their own kind of battle
Remember to be nice always
We can often underestimate the power of a
simple
'Hi, how are you?'

I believe the very first sign of a problem in my brain might have started as far back as 1995 when I went on my own to visit my brother Tom while he was working in Jersey. I stayed for a week and each day while he was at work, I would go on the various day trips available for tourists like myself.

On one of these excursions I travelled by boat and then bus to a little village market situated in the North of France. While I was checking out these markets, something happened inside my brain. It's difficult to explain, but suddenly I felt this weird reverberation, something like I have now with LBD but much, much worse. All of a sudden, I was unable to see properly, I was unable to walk properly nor was I able to communicate with anyone. I remember thinking, if I could only get back to the bus and sit down I might be OK, but this feeling in my brain went on for what seemed like an eternity. There and then I was convinced that there was something seriously wrong with my brain, but I had no idea what it was.

I was trying to compose myself, while at the same time getting more terrified because here I was in the North of France, completely alone and was thinking, how am I going to get out of here?

My head was spinning and if I moved it, I felt my brain float and follow a second later. I remember holding onto the stall nearest to me and using it for support as I tried to walk in the direction of the bus. I soon learned that I wasn't able to focus enough to even know which direction the bus was in. I stood there holding on for dear life to the stall and rooted to the ground but thankfully after a few minutes, my sight seemed to be getting a little better.

Once that happened I was able to slowly get my bearings and headed towards the bus. As I made my way back I noticed that with every step I took, I could feel the pressure applied to the ground with my shoe being echoed in my brain. I eventually made it to the bus by holding onto whatever I could. Even though no one asked me if I was alright, I clearly recall people looking at me with what seemed to be expressions of concern. I really felt that I must have looked like I was having a stroke. I clambered onto the bus and drank some water. As I began to relax with relief in the comfort of the bus, all the bad feelings I had in my head seemed to fade away and my eyesight started to come back to normal.

By the time I got back to Jersey that evening, I was feeling good again and decided not to say anything to anyone because I knew if Tom found out about this incident, he would insist I go to the hospital and then my holiday would indeed be ruined and anyway I was feeling fine again. To this day I never found out the reason why my brain went into overload that day, but I do remember being nervous on my own for a long time afterwards. Looking back now, it was foolish of me not to seek medical advice when I returned home but I was only in my early 30s and of course believed I was invincible.

What effect did this episode have on my health?

Chapter Four

My blood pressure, was that how it all started?

I have always considered myself a 'strong' man however I truly realise my strength when being 'strong' is my only option.

My second trip to hospital was in 1999.

This time at St Marys' Orthopaedic in Cork having an operation on a prolapsed disc. I had been suffering quite a lot with back pain which is a common side effect of working on building sites, but this pain was on another level. It was totally different and was self-inflicted, I can still remember exactly the day and time that I damaged it. I lifted the hitch of a heavy trailer off the back of a jeep by myself as I was in too much of a hurry to ask for help. At that time, I had my own building company and I was laid up for a couple of months thanks to this back injury. This led to keyhole surgery which the surgeon said was successful but because I didn't follow the advice of my doctor and allow time for recovery, I ended up back in hospital twice within a couple of months having two separate epidurals in my back to relieve the severe pain.

When I went back to work I was becoming stressed out by the workload, I could have delegated the duties as I had 45 people employed in my building company but unfortunately, I didn't. I was beginning to attend my doctor possibly every two weeks with different symptoms, headaches, dizzy spells, anxiety and just a general feeling of being unwell.

On one of these visits around 2002, he told me that my blood pressure was at a high level and needed further checking in hospital. Helena took me to Cork and I was admitted to hospital and my stay lasted for 18 days. I didn't feel too bad lying down, even though my Blood Pressure was up and down a lot, but the very minute I would stand up or get out of bed I would collapse needing assistance. It took about ten days before I could go to the bathroom unaided. After many tests including checking for blockages to my heart, the results came back, and all was clear. On discharge, I was given blood pressure medications and aspirin etc. but was taken off the aspirin a couple of years ago, having been on it for fourteen years.

For a few years afterwards, my blood pressure fluctuated a lot and at one time I was on four different tablets to keep it in control. Every now and then I would be given the 24-hour monitor with varying results and by then my sleep patterns were all over the place, bad but not quite as bad as they are now. I would just be exhausted in the early afternoon and nod off so easily but then spend most nights twisting and turning getting no proper night time sleep whatsoever. Upon reflection I feel that a lot of my problems including the blood pressure was exasperated by stress. Even if I went away for a weekend with Helena I would also bring along worry about the upcoming week, the next job, when the next cheque was due to me or when the next big bill was due to be paid.

Here I felt I was on a merry-go-round and this was the one for the big boys and one I was not too comfortable to be a part of. I would love to tell you that it is wonderful being self-employed, but I learned that it is not all it's cracked up to be. My health suffered, and I honestly believe that my brain didn't get a moments' quiet or down time for years. It didn't take long before I started getting chest pain and finding it quite hard to breathe. I was taken to Mallow A & E, where they did all the necessary tests, the tracing of my heart appeared ok and I was advised I could go home. Later that evening I got a call from the hospital asking me to come back the following morning at 10 am. I was doing a job in Charleville with my brother Tom and went to work as usual at 8 am and went from there to the hospital at the appointed time.

When I arrived at the hospital, to say they were making a fuss of me would be an understatement as I was met with a multitude of questions asking how I was feeling, any chest pain etc. Apparently, the result of the blood tests showed that some enzymes were out of sync and they were concerned in case I had already suffered a mild heart attack. Fortunately, all was OK, I was feeling fine and went back to work.

From then on, every now and then I would get chest pain, sometimes worse than others with a tightness in my chest. I had a path worn to my GP and thankfully each time I was given the all clear. The great thing to come out of this trip to Mallow hospital was that I gave up smoking. Also, the look on Tom's face when I came back from hospital and started to smoke again, I could see he was genuinely worried and this just made it easier for me to quit smoking. I had been a smoker for approximately 20 years, not a very heavy smoker around 20 a day. I found it difficult but when I had a craving I would have a light cigar and eventually had to wean myself off of them - no weaning needed off the bottle, I gave up the beer in 1990 and didn't have another for 11 years.

A problem arose for me after giving up the cigarettes, I gained weight, a lot of weight. I was always around fourteen to fourteen and a half stone, but within two years I was knocking on the door of twenty stone. More chest pain, more doctors' visits, more hospital visits, stress tests - you name it. Around the same time, I completed a Diploma Course in the Psychology Department in UCC. I learned so much from this course and in many ways, it changed my life, it changed how I looked at life in general and my whole approach to life.

In 2006 I decided I had to do something about my weight and started choosing healthier options in my diet on a daily basis and at the same time started walking a little, easy does it, when I saw an advertisement for a charity walk to Machu Picchu in South America and I was hooked. I got all the details, filled out the necessary forms and from then on, I got serious about my lifestyles changes including the walking and from then on, I called it trek training. It was a ten-day trek and you had to be pretty fit for it. I gave up potatoes and bread and was soon walking five miles twice a day and honestly it did me good.

We were trekking at a very high altitude, the air was very light and there were times when I found it difficult to breathe. During that trip I had a few dizzy spells, but felt the cause was due to the lack of oxygen which is common. The group I went with were fantastic and they made the difficult trek a wonderful unforgettable experience. When I arrived home, every meal was accompanied by either bread or spuds but thankfully my hunger for such a diet didn't last very long.

Chapter Five

One of the biggest steps in my life

When I look back on how far I have come since my diagnosis, I realise that steps I considered to be small have actually been steps of most significance.

From 2006 to 2010 life was very much a roller coaster as far as my health was concerned.

I was forced to close my building company and it broke my heart. It was hard times, hard to collect money owed and I basically never got paid for some work. That in itself brought on a lot of stress again and as a follow up more chest pain, more hospital visits and more sleepless nights.

Always in a hurry, I suppose trying to get ahead of the stress there was one evening I didn't even give myself time to eat my dinner properly. I obviously tried to swallow a sizable chunk of a roast potato, potatoes seem to be my downfall and unfortunately this roasting hot roast potato got lodged in my throat. I reacted instantly and coughed it out with such force that I added fuel to fire. I knew instantly by the pain that something was wrong, and my throat was not only burnt but worse. Once again, I went straight to Mallow A & E where I had to spend the following three nights recuperating as my throat had begun to swell and close up. I was told to take time to chew my food really well in future and in actual fact to follow the rule *'eat your liquids and drink your food'*.

Not one to stay down, I started up another business, this time a fitted furniture company and business was going great until I started taking on big jobs like schemes of houses from big builders and big developers. I had once again found myself on the big boys' merry-go-round, trying to collect money owed for the jobs and it wasn't long before I had all the usual headaches back again.

In October 2009 my stepson Shane got married to a beautiful Australian girl called Jessica. We travelled to their wedding in Sydney and had a wonderful time with the family and could clearly see that the economy there was much better than at home. While we were there, we decided that as there was a down turn at home, with the Celtic tiger already on its' last legs, it might be a good time to take the bull by the horns and move to the sunny Southern Hemisphere. By this time I was 45 years old and thankfully secured a work visa for Australia. I fitted the necessary criteria and this visa also allowed Helena permission to work there.

At that time, the economy in Ireland was collapsing, work was drying up, the bills were piling up, the banks were squeezing everyone, and we figured there was more to gain than lose. I didn't want to look back in ten years' time and have regrets for not making the move to Australia, fair enough if it didn't work out but with Helena by my side all would be well. Most of our friends believed we were mad to be taking on such a big move at this time of our lives, but funny thing, when we came back on holiday twelve months later they all agreed that we were dead right to have made the move when we did and felt we must have had a premonition on how really bad Irelands' economy was going to get.

Having made that decision, it wasn't so difficult saying goodbye to the family in Australia in November after the wedding, as we knew that we would be seeing them all again very soon but leaving Ireland with sad goodbyes would be another matter entirely.

We arrived home on a mission and booked our tickets for Australia, confirming that we were leaving Ireland on Valentines' Day, February 14th, 2010. We had so much to do in the intervening time to get organised and had a great Christmas as the newly- weds were home and my son Pat had a beautiful little baby girl called Hollie just before Christmas, therefore lots of reasons for celebrations. By now our children were grown up and my three step children were in Sydney, but my own children were still in Ireland.

When Women's Christmas, January 6th rolled around, I felt the date for our departure was coming all too soon and the reality of leaving was beginning to sink in. I discussed the move with my kids and their response was enthusiastic, telling us that when we were settled they would probably follow us. I am so thankful that this is exactly what happened. We got a lovely apartment right across from the beach in the Sydney suburb of Cronulla just up the street from where we stayed when out for the wedding but this time we were not on holidays. Before long we were both working, I was on the buildings and Helena had secured a position in an office in Sydneys' City centre, we were living in a beautiful place which added to our lovely lifestyle.

I believe this major change of address is one of the main reasons that I'm alive today. A couple of months before we went to the wedding in Australia, the pressure of losing my business once again was getting to me and I felt it was just the last straw. I went into the 40ft metal container that was at the back of the garden, put a rope around my neck and was going to end it all, but for some reason, don't know why, but at that moment 'reason' broke through and asked me the question, how could I do this to Helena and the children?

Thankfully, I changed my mind.

By moving to Australia, I felt in a way that I would be leaving my bad luck behind me, hopefully get my health back on track and of course the icing on the cake – better weather!

Chapter Six
More hospital visits

I have been knocked down

I have had to build on my self preservation and strength on a daily basis – my mental health care requires the same amount of effort as lifting weights at the gym!

As I said in the last chapter leaving the children and our beautiful Granddaughter Hollie was very difficult. Thankfully and gradually over the next twelve to eighteen months one by one they all came to Australia to give it a try, knowing that when we were there they would be safe and had a home to go to. We were so excited each time going to the airport to pick them up, especially the day that little Hollie arrived. I can still feel the excitement inside me as I write, that is such a fond memory.

Celebrating our second Christmas in Sydney was a pure delight for the soul, as we had dinner on the balcony of our apartment with the table set for fifteen which comprised of my beautiful wife, our six children and their partners, Hollie and a few relatives. Now that was a wonderful day and we had a very Merry Christmas at the other side of the world - blessed to have all our family around us.

It wasn't until the following year on a trip back to Ireland that it struck me what a special Christmas that really was. I called to see my Uncle Joe and his beautiful wife Theresa, who at the time was very ill with cancer but she had said that under no circumstances was I to go back to Australia without saying goodbye.

This was going to be a particularly sad goodbye for all three of us as I believe Joe, Theresa and myself knew that it was likely I would not see her again. In fact that was the case as sadly Theresa passed away three months after my visit. Without doubt one of the nicest things anyone had ever said to me is what Theresa said to me that day and I quote, *'Kev you must have been a great Dad because they all wound up outside in Australia with you'*. To this day I often think about it because being a Father who was separated you often wonder how good or bad a Dad you have been, but at least in Theresa's eyes I was a good one! Thank you, Theresa.

In Sydney I needed to have a GP to write up prescriptions for my blood pressure medicines etc. and while the place is full of medical centres, I was very lucky to find a doctor who ran his own practice just down the street from where I lived. He was like a doctor in a country practice in Ireland, in that we became good friends and he didn't have to look at the file to know who I was. Over time he changed some of my medication, tried some others, motivated me to lose some weight and eat a healthier diet. It was easy and soon I started feeling better, I loved to swim in the ocean or take walks on the beach and believe it or not, I actually did catch a wave or two.

Every now and again my blood pressure would go out of control and I could be out of work sometimes for a few weeks at a time, even on a couple of occasions ending up in hospital. I really believed that living near the beach in Sydney with fresh air and lots of exercise was the key to better health for me.

I also had three serious stays in hospital while in Sydney, the first of which happened around 1am on a Monday morning. I got up to use the toilet and while I was going back to bed I suddenly got a most awful pain in my chest. It was terrible, and I called Helena and told her I was in trouble. She said she would drive me to hospital but then it became clear that I needed an Ambulance. When the medics arrived, they checked me out and said I was most likely having a heart attack and started there and then treating me for it. I remember one of the crew saying, 'Stay with us Kevin' and I was thinking to myself this cannot be good. I was rushed off to Sutherland Hospital which was only ten minutes away and on arrival I was put on all the monitors once again, had many tests and was given some more pain relief which I needed badly.

To everyones surprise the tracing of the heart seemed to be OK, no trace of a heart attack but everything else suggested I was having a heart attack. They tried a different machine, same result, but yet all the signs were there. When the blood results came back they showed no sign of a heart attack either. I still had severe chest pain and felt very sick. There was one particular doctor who was about to finish her shift but told us that she was going nowhere 'till she and her team found out what was wrong as she would have to solve this conundrum. She returned after about two hours and said that she was pretty sure they had found the cause of my problem.

I had contracted a disease called **Coxsackie Virus** otherwise known as **Bornholm Disease** or more commonly called **The Devils Grip** because of the pain and the way it can mimic the symptoms of a heart attack. Trust me, the Devils Grip is a very good name for it and I would say pretty apt. Now at least they knew what I had, they could start treatment. The following morning the specialist came to see me only to tell me, that I was the only patient he had seen with Devils Grip in the hospital in over 15 years. In fact, it was so uncommon that most of his staff would never even have heard of it, but for the investigative work that fine lady doctor had done, God only knows what would have happened. I spent a week in hospital and it was a couple more weeks before I got my strength up enough to be able to return to work.

Chapter Seven
True friends are invaluable

Thankfully no matter whether I was in Ireland or Australia I was always surrounded by great friends – not a bad complaint to have!

Time was moving on in Australia, and my brother Tom, his wife and family emmigrated from Ireland to live in Perth. Even though it's a about a six-hour flight from Sydney to Perth, it felt great knowing my brother was in the same country. Tom like his wife as you will see in a later chapter has always been brilliant to me and especially now that I have LBD.

My 50th Birthday was coming up on September 9th, 2013 and we decided to have a big party. I ended up in hospital again while planning for the party, this time with high blood pressure but thankfully I wasn't there long just two nights and was back home and well just a couple of weeks before the party.

My Dad and Mam along with two of their friends flew out from Ireland. I got a lovely shock when my brother Liam who was on business in the Philippines flew in to surprise me, I was both delighted and surprised to see him. My brother in law Dave flew from Melbourne and my wonderful friend Mary from Brisbane. I had close to one hundred guests but most important of all was the moment when the photo was taken with myself, Helena and our six children, life was wonderful.

My parents were flying back home from Perth, so we all had a lovely holiday in Perth with Tom, his wife Julie and family before they left for home. Again, we had to say our goodbyes, which I absolutely hate. It reminds me of the feelings I had when saying goodbye to my Grandparents when they died. I think... Is this it, what if I never see them again like at a funeral when you know... This is it. All the celebrations are over, back to work and weeks pass, the weather is beautiful because it is now October and I am facing into Summer in Sydney with an air of optimism.

Out of the blue, one morning as I was getting ready for work I felt I had a cold, runny nose, bit of a cough and a slight headache, but I didn't think much of it. Even if I had been very sick I couldn't miss work as I was site manager on a big apartment block and I had a site meeting called for 1 o'clock. I arrived at the site as usual at 6.45am to get things ready and got myself a hot coffee. I began to feel worse as the morning was going on, and I knew I must have looked as bad as I felt when my boss came in and said, *'my God Kev are you*

OK, you don't look so good', I replied it's only a head cold.

At around midday I was getting worse and feeling terrible, to the point that he told me to go home but I wouldn't go because of our 1 o'clock meeting. This meeting had just begun when my vision started to get blurred and even though on that day the temperature was in the low 30s, I was freezing. I excused myself and left for home as at this stage everyone could see how sick I was. Then I proceeded to do one of the most stupid things I had ever done in my life. I was not fit to drive but I drove home through Sydney traffic. There I was all rugged up like forty coats, the heater turned onto the last and still shivering.

This drive from hell took about an hour and to this day, I really don't know how I made it home alive and didn't crash into any poor innocent motorist. When I got there my hands were so cold I found it difficult to put the key in the lock and I was very glad there was a lift in that apartment. I then rang Helena who was at work and she told me that she would leave the office straight away and for me to go to bed. When Helena arrived, she took one look at me and called an Ambulance again.

The medics arrived and as I had the blinds closed they turned on the bedroom light but had to turn it off again as it was hurting my eyes. I was put into the Ambulance without delay with a towel over my head to shield me from the light and off to Sutherland Hospital once more. As I was stretchered off the Ambulance at the hospital I'm glad to say my sense of humour was still intact as I heard a lady say out loud to the crew….. *Is he dead?* to which I answered….*I hope not.* A long evening and night of pain and sickness ensued, and the staff tried their best to give me some relief with different medications.

One of the doctors tried on four occasions to do a lumbar puncture to they take fluid from my spine to confirm Viral Meningitis as they had already started to treat me for it. I found this to be a very painful procedure and four different times he had the needle inserted and for some reason or other he was unable to get any fluid. On that fourth and final occasion I told him in no uncertain terms, that was it, I will die before I will let you do that again, as a result I didn't forget that doctor for a long time.

For a few months before that I had noticed every now and then I would get a sharp pain in my right hip, especially if I was getting in or out of a truck or climbing a ladder but I thought to myself that I was far too young to be having hip problems. I didn't mention it to anyone as I was afraid that if I did, a hip operation might be on the cards.

Then one day while still in hospital recovering, I was getting out of bed and I let out a little moan, the nurse present asked if I was OK and I explained my case to her. A short time later a doctor came in and examined me, moving my hip and leg this way and that. Even though she did this in a very gentle manner I found it terribly painful. Within a couple of hours, I was wheeled off for what they called a Nuclear Scan, they not only scanned my hip but my whole body. Australia's Health Service were fantastic, not only were they very quick to respond, but I was never in a waiting room for long and were also very thorough.

The following morning two lovely Doctors came into my room and told me that the results were back. I had Paget's Disease of the Bone, to which I responded, 'Oh Thank God'.

The lady doctor looked surprised and said do you know about it as we don't really, while holding her iPhone up telling me that they both had to research it. I replied 'never heard of it doctor but at least now I know I have not been imagining the pain'. The doctor proceeded to tell me that it was considered an English disease and as there is obviously a high population of English people in Australia it was common many years ago, but now considered rare.

I'm the type of person that when something is wrong I want to know as much information as possible. I found out that Paget's Disease of the Bone interferes with the body's' normal recycling process, in which new bone tissue gradually replaces the old bone tissue. Over time this disease can cause the affected bones to become fragile and misshapen. This most commonly occurs in the pelvis, spine and legs. Complications of this disease can include broken bones, back pain and hip pain. This can also lead to hearing loss or headaches if the skull is affected.

My own GP in Cronulla compared it to concrete explaining there is sand, cement and stone in concrete and if you have too much stone in the concrete it makes the mix weak. That is what this disease does, it mixes a bad batch of bone. I won't say too much more about it, but it played a big part in trying to discover what was wrong before I was diagnosed with LBD. I sometimes worry about it, as at times my balance is not good and if I fall and break a bone it could lead to complications, but more about that later.

I was in hospital on this occasion for 16 nights and this stay took a lot out of me. It took me about 6 months to recover fully. I had regular follow up appointments with my fantastic GP in Cronulla. I also had many appointments in the hospital as I was told I had Paget's disease in my hip and skull and the Specialist was particularly interested in the fact that I had bone malformations in my mouth and jaw.

I had finished up my job as site manager as it was a very physically as well as mentally challenging, but I did a few hours' work driving a machine to help a few people out but to be fair I didn't do much as I wasn't really able. If I worked for a few hours on any given day, it would take me days to recover, so looking back on it I wasn't totally surprised with what my doctor was about to tell me.

Towards what I thought was the end of my recovery, Helena had attended my GP with me and told me that I ought to think long and hard about my future as he said my career in construction as over, as far as what I was doing anyway, climbing scaffolding, up and down ladders, walking over rough ground on building sites and regularly getting in and out of trucks or machines. As I was hands on in my job, staying put was not an option and I placed complete trust in the good GP. Both Helena and I went for a coffee to the little coffee place right on the edge of the beach and discussed what he had said. I have to say I was a little sad about it but had to face up to the fact that this chapter of my life was now finished but as always in my life another chapter was about to begin.

Having spent most of my life in construction and sales, but mainly construction I would find it difficult to make a change. I had a great job as site manager of an apartment block with a basement car park, four shops, fifty four apartments and two penthouses overlooking the Sydney Harbour Bridge. I had the complete running of the site and even though at times it was challenging, it was also mentally rewarding with great job satisfaction. The architectural drawings alone for a job this size didn't even phase me. I knew that I had come a long way through hard work, study, a little luck and sheer determination. I had worked my way up to a very good position that paid well and having to give it up was not easy to take.

I decided to go back to sales and within a matter of days I got a job designing and selling kitchens. I was excited to attend a two-week training programme and when completed I hit the ground running. On my first day the office had arranged 3 appointments for me, 10am, 2pm & 7pm and on my second call at 2pm I sold a kitchen and would sell at least one a day. They were long days, but the wages reflected that.

Around that time, I was beginning to accept the fact that I would not be returning to full health therefore Helena and I started talking about the possibility of buying a little house in Ireland just in case my health went from bad to worse. House prices had fallen significantly back home and even though we were keeping a watchful eye on the internet this notion was only a plan for the future at this stage as we were both very happy in Australia. We now had a second grandchild as Shane and Jessica had a beautiful boy called Charlie.

Now and then I would have to take time off work due to a whole host of different symptoms. I was beginning to notice at times my balance wasn't right. Sometimes I had blurred vision and found it difficult to focus. My hearing would be good one day and very bad another.

My blood pressure problems had returned and it was very erratic. The company I worked for understood and were very accommodating as they could see I had a pattern of ill health. When feeling well I could work long hours and sell seven plus kitchens per week, but then before long I would feel sick again, take time off and when rested for a few days I would be good to go again.

Chapter Eight
My angels keep watch

Angel of God, my guardian dear
To whom God's love, commits me here
Ever this day, be at my side
To light and guard, to rule and guide
Amen

At 1.50am one Monday morning, as my brother Tom says, I got the phone call from home that you dread when you are so far away, and these calls always seem to come in the middle of the night. It was my brother Liam calling to say that Dad was in hospital in Limerick having had a stroke. To be fair to Liam, this mustn't have been easy for him either trying to tell us how bad Dad was without worrying us too much, but it was obvious that it was pretty serious.

We flew home, and it was only then we realised just how unwell he had been and what a tough time Mam and the rest of the family had gone through. They were advised to tell Dad that we were coming home because if we just walked in on him it might set him back. We went in and gave him a big hug and at least he still had his sense of humour as the first thing he said was…. *'God everyone will say he's very bad, the boys are home from Australia'*. Tom's wife Julie came home with us and as a nurse she was a brilliant help, especially when it came to organising the rehab for Dad in the hospital that she had worked in previously.

We had seen a house on the internet for sale and while at home I went to have a look at it. It was very good value and having decided to buy it, I put down a deposit. We said our goodbyes to Dad and all the family and said would be seeing them all again early in the New Year.

Early September I arrived back in Sydney, but it took me longer than usual to get over the effects of the trip. I went back to work and very soon started to feel unwell again, a lot of hip pain, blurred vision, balance and blood pressure problems, pretty much more of the same. I knew I would have to make changes once again and I got a new job with less hours, working for a small family business with a massive reputation. I worked a salesman designing bedroom units, wardrobes and shower screens. The company owners were Sam and Marissa DiMartino, who were fantastic and I am still in touch with. It was my dream job. I would start work at 9am, do six pre-appointed calls and sometimes I was home at lunchtime. Out of the six calls I was selling an average of four to five and on a great day even six. Yes, I was a good salesman, had a good rapport with the customers but most important of all Sam and Marissa were brilliant at what they did, ran a beautiful organisation and treated each customer like they were royalty. It was the most well-paid job I ever had and I loved it.

Things were looking up again, the news from Dad was good and thank god he had made a full recovery. Helena and I had decided to go home after Christmas but pushed the date out to February and the best deal on the tickets happened to be on Valentine's Day.

Maybe a little serendipitous as it was on February 14^{th,} that we left Ireland exactly five years before.

At this stage I thought of it as a bit romantic and another little adventure and believed we would get the new house sorted out, do some badly needed work on it and then return to Australia after a few months. But not for the first time, that is not the way it turned out because my life would take another twist.

My job was going really well and as we had a lot of nice stuff gathered in the five years as well of a lot of tools therefore we made arrangement to ship them home and they would get there around the same time as ourselves. All was well as Helena and I had made this decision together and to say that she is the love of my life is putting it mildly as she is simply my rock.

The kids were happy all doing their own thing, had beautiful Grandchildren, just bought a little cottage in Ireland, selling wardrobes left, right and centre, making good money and looking forward to Christmas which in Australia is the big summer holiday time. Just after Christmas we spent a week in Melbourne with my brother in law Dave, who was recuperating having had major heart surgery. We stayed with him for a week and as was usual on all our visits with him, we had a right royal auld time.

When we returned to Sydney I noticed that there was a three-day cruise, something we had always planned to do in the preceding five years but just never got around to it. As we got on board this massive cruise liner, 16 decks high I remember both of us looking at each other and laughing as all the other boats in the water seemed so small in comparison. As we sailed out under Sydney Harbour Bridge in glowing sunshine to the sound of the ship's horn, my arm around the love of my life and a bottle of cold beer in the other I thought the worst is over. The music played as the sun went down on the most beautiful harbour in the World. It was one of the happiest times of my life. I felt alive, I felt healthier than I had in a long time, I was also delighted that Helena was getting a much needed break because when I've been sick, she's always there to pick up the pieces which can't be easy.

Back to work again with only a few weeks to go before leaving for home, but alas my health was once more going to come against me. I had bad chest pain one night while at the same time finding it very hard to breathe. I felt so sick that I knew I was unable to travel by car to the hospital so once again Helena called an Ambulance. I was again whisked off to Sutherland Hospital only this time there seemed to be a lot more panic with everyone. I was wheeled into a room and the staff were doing their thing as usual with wires and needles when I heard over the loud speaker system.... *'Doctors to resus one, Doctors to resus one'*... thinking O' Dear God, there must be some patient in bigger trouble than myself........ just then my eyes were drawn to a sign up on the wall which read ... RESUS 1 Ooops! They were being called for me.

I seemed to be drifting in and out of consciousness and all I can remember is finding it so hard to breathe even with the oxygen mask on. I was eventually stabilized and given high doses of pain killers, the pain in my chest felt like someone had stuck a knife in me and was twisting it every time I moved. Even when I was put on the vaporised form of Ventolin it hurt so much to even breathe that in and that pain continued for a couple of days. I remember the Doctor coming into me one morning when I was eventually out of danger and he was smiling. I asked him ….what are you smiling at? and he answered saying that he and his colleague were wondering how I was this morning and when they got to about 7 metres from the ward, he could hear me breathing and they said to each other…'that answers that'.

This time I was diagnosed with the H5N1 Virus known as Bird Flu. The Doctor told me that while this can vary in humans from a range of typical flu symptoms like sore throat, muscle pain or pneumonia, I had developed quite a number of severe symptoms. He said I was lucky that Helena called the Ambulance when she did as I was treated by the good doctors and nurses in the nick of time. He couldn't confirm where I picked it up but surmised that it may have been from a sea gull as I lived close to the beach.

I spent another two weeks in hospital and at one stage the doctors told me that it was too early to say whether I would be allowed to fly home on February 14th or not. During this time, we spoke about the fact that this trip home may not only be for a couple of months but may be time to move home for good.

The morning I was being discharged my doctor came to the ward to have a chat with both of us and we were told that the doctors had a patient conference on me to discuss the fact that I had Coxsackie Virus, Viral Meningitis, Paget's Disease and now H5N1 all happening within a relatively short period of time. He first wanted to know our future plans and I told him that due to my poor health we had planned to move back home to Ireland.

That day I will never forget the longest day I'll live. The doctor said and I thought it was very well put....'that for His Peace of Mind and he hoped that he was wrong and was probably wrong but when I get back to Ireland I should have myself checked out for Parkinson's Disease or Dementia'. I already had one Uncle in Australia who had passed away from Parkinson's and my Uncle Dave who I mentioned earlier was at that time struggling with his battle against Alzheimer's.

I was in shock, only 51 years of age and I felt like I was at the beginning of possibly the biggest fight of my life. I looked at Helena and I knew by her expression that she felt the same.

I was discharged from hospital and would never again work in Australia. I had a follow up appointment with my lovely GP in Cronulla and he agreed with the doctors in the Hospital. I found out that he had taken a personal interest in my medical history and each time I was in hospital he had been personally in touch with my doctors. I got such brilliant care in Southerland hospital and for that I am very grateful.

Finally an end comes to our wonderful adventure in Australia.

Chapter Nine
Survival

I didn't choose the word survival lightly for this chapter as honestly it is the only way to describe what I am going through, with the help of my family & friends I am surviving.

I will continue where I left off in the next section because of the title Lewy Body Dementia, Survival and Me and because the end of my story, is really not the end of my story, but more the beginning of my journey with LBD.

I have given you a brief description of the kind of person I am and how lucky I am to have such a wonderful wife, 3 children Noreen, Pat and Kevin and 3 step children Declan, Shane and Michelle. Also, at the time of writing I have four gorgeous Grandchildren, Hollie, Charlie, Liam and Victoria, two in Sydney and two in Ireland.

Please remember, this is my journey and first of all I would like to bring you along this path as I see it from and secondly my biggest wish is that this may be of help to you or a loved one, even if it's only to open the door to a conversation about the difficult subject of suicide. I cannot stress enough that the things I talk about are either about myself or my thoughts on things that have influenced me in my life and in no way do I intend to upset or cause offence to anyone and I do not offer any medical advice. I am just an ordinary person suffering from the horrible disease LBD.

If you think something is bothering someone…….
Ask the question, **how are you feeling**….

Ask **is everything alright**…. some might say, yes everything is fine……but then that's your chance to listen, if someone doesn't want to talk and you know there is something wrong, tell them that you are there if they need you.

Some people have bad days and some people have bad lives and by that, I mean on this occasion inside their heads. If you bottle up all of the small things, then the tree begins to grow, and it soon gets out of hand. For me, I found that if I could really talk about what was going on, believe me it helped a lot.

The thing is we never know what happens behind closed doors, nor do we know what happens in the hidden mind. Why not knock gently on those doors by sharing a smile, maybe even complementing them on some achievement no matter how small, or how they look or something personal to them.

This might actually just be enough for them to return your smile and remember your smile is worth nothing 'till you give it away and then it's priceless and eventually the person may trust you enough to talk.

Chapter Ten
To every parent their newborn baby is just perfect

I am so lucky to be surrounded by amazing family and friends. They remind me every day how lucky I am, how loved I am and despite my illness how much I have to be grateful for.

As I mentioned previously I spent a little time studying and I remember doing work on the following statement *'every baby born is 100% perfect'* that includes you, me and every single person around us.

I agree with this statement and as new babies are taught to do nearly everything, this learnt behaviour is all important. Our babies are so beautiful and a lot of work but even at the best of times parenting can be challenging. We as parents sometimes over protect, in that in todays' world we don't like to see our children lose at anything or feeling hurt and we want them to believe that good will always happen. Wrong.

We are not doing them justice. I am not saying to tell an eight-year-old the full effects of LBD - actually that very thing brings to mind the Crystal Project in Mallow, Ireland who brought out a wonderful book called **'Feathers in my brain'.**
This really lovely book helps children in a lovely gentle way to understand dementia. It is perfectly acceptable to say Grandanz (as my Granddaughter calls me) is sick and also to be on the losing team at a match, or maybe not in the running for medals at Irish dancing or even losing out at a County Final. All of these are

part of life and almost essential training for the future to let them see that things will get better, it might take some time to get over losing but it will happen, and things will get better.

When you lose at something the first couple of times don't give up because when you eventually win, it makes winning all the sweeter. When I was on the pitch myself I remember I'd be told to 'lick your wounds and move on'. That may have been a bit harsh, but I think the best way is somewhere in the middle.

What I am trying to say is to love your family unconditionally and be there for them, protect them from all harm at all costs but it's important for them to know that things will not always go their own way.

There will be times they will feel pain, sometimes terrible pain in their lives and when they do they will hopefully talk about it and ask for help. Keeping things bottled up is not good because eventually the bottle will burst.

The day I was diagnosed with LBD which I will go into later, I asked the doctor what to expect and asked if some information on it could be posted to me. As I told you before I'm the kind who wants to know everything.

Helena and I left the Neurologist's office, headed home and spoke about it for days. I researched it on the internet and while it can be a very good source of information, it can also 'diagnose' you with a number of ailments that you apparently have, and you can quickly get sucked down that rabbit hole.

I was delighted to receive the correct information from my doctor in relation to my diagnosis. It definitely took a few months before it hit me as to what exactly the doctor had really said and how serious a diagnosis it was. One of the doctors suggested to me to note my symptoms on a daily basis as they were so varied and that suggestion was the catalyst for writing this book. Never in a million years, did I ever think I could write a book and although writing it has brought back many painful memories, I feel that it's good for my brain to have a focus. I have joined and become part of lots of societies on social media like the LBD organizations and survival groups and find them all so helpful.

Chapter Eleven
Searching for hope

I firmly believe that what I am going through now is a true test from the man above, I may not understand why I am going though it now, but I know that someday I will.

To be honest when we moved back to Ireland I was feeling good again, not too concerned with my health as I felt the worst was over and it was the beginning of a new adventure again for myself and Helena.

The house that we had put the deposit on didn't work out and as it happened we bought a beautiful little place out the country where we live today, and we called it 'Rose Cottage'.

I started working for myself and in my mind all that I needed was enough work to bring in a decent wage every week, I no longer had any interest in building up a business again. Australia had been good to us and I just wanted enough to keep going. After a few months I was finding it more difficult to do any type of physical work, not that I wasn't able, but I was just under pressure as I had pains everywhere but especially in my right shoulder.

I made an appointment to see the GP who had access to all my old medical records and told him all about the health issues I encountered while I was away. I told him that the doctor in Australia had said to get checked for early onset Parkinson's and Alzheimer's. He wrote to the Neurologist requesting an appointment for me and I was called to see the Neurologist in November 2015.

In the meantime, having been self-employed for seven months, I decided to give up working for myself and got a job as a salesman in September 2015 which I must say I enjoyed very much, but again there were days where my energy levels were so low and all I wanted to do was sleep.

Trying to concentrate would at times prove very difficult, even though I was designing kitchens and it was a job I loved and was good at - I knew something was wrong because I could make silly mistakes. I would spot them, but I was still making them, and this began to frustrate me. I might have an appointment to meet a customer and would take the wrong road and if I didn't write everything down I could forget appointments, dates, directions, people's names, but for my diary I could remember nothing and sometimes I would even forget to write things down.

My writing was getting worse and sometimes I had a little tremor in my left hand and when lying down my right leg had a mind of its' own and would go into pretty much a constant tremor. The neurologist made an appointment for me to have a Lumbar Puncture two weeks after my first visit. The week after my lumbar puncture I started to build a small workshop at home. I was doing it in the evenings and on weekends, but it was taking me ten times longer to do it than it normally should. My energy levels were at an all-time low and it would be the last big job that I would ever do. The company that I was working for at the time seemed happy with me and I stayed working with them until Christmas 2015.

I was sick over Christmas even though I had lots of time to rest. I discussed it with my doctor and told him that I just wasn't feeling right, I felt my head was all over the place and I basically couldn't trust myself to do my job the way it was supposed to be done and I had to be fair to the company as well.

My doctor agreed on examination of my symptoms and it was decided that I could no longer work. I had very mixed feelings because deep down I knew that something was very wrong but there was relief also because the pressure of the job was now gone. I was called back to see my neurologist in February 2016 as she had the results of the Lumbar Puncture and it was on that visit I was told that it looked like I had Parkinson's. I was examined by two doctors that day and gave them all of my symptoms which I will go into later. It was frightening to be told this but on the other hand again there was a bit of relief in that it explained what was wrong with me. The neurologist ordered different bloods to be taken and also an MRI Scan. I was rescheduled to go back to see her in a couple of months but in the meantime the pain in my hips was beginning to be unbearable, so bad that I could only walk with the aid of a walking frame. As a result, I had a path worn to my GP getting different pain killers, but nothing seemed to be working.

I then got an appointment to see an orthopaedic surgeon and after some more tests and scans he didn't seem to think that Paget's disease was the cause of my excessive hip pain that radiated across my lower back. The results of X-rays and CT scans were clear only showing up normal wear and tear, which he said was common for one such as I who worked in the buildings all my life. I was then given Butrans patches 5mg for the pain and they would over a short period of time be increased to 30mg. They went a long way in getting rid of the excruciating pain but only over the course of about twelve months.

For my next two visits to my neurologist I would attend walking as I said with the aid of a walking frame.

On one of my first visits I was asked if I had any funny kinds of dreams or nightmares and the answer is yes. I will explain as I need to dedicate one whole chapter to my dreams or should I say nightmares. I always discussed them with Helena, they were so real that it was like I was living in two different worlds. The next couple of months would prove to be particularly challenging and again I had cause to visit my GP very regularly. I have to say that I was feeling pretty low and as I said in constant pain. I was put on anti-depressants and started to see a psychiatrist. The visits to the psychiatrist were every six weeks but there was something that was not sitting right with me and after four or five visits I didn't return to see him anymore.

On a visit to my neurologist in February 2017 all of the symptoms that I had were still there and some were even worse and there were some new ones to be added to the list. One of them that comes to mind is waking up at night for no particular reason and breaking into what I think was something like hot flushes. I could go from being very hot to very cold in a matter of five minutes and this could happen a couple of times a night and of course no reprieve from the pain.

Pain, pain and more pain.

Chapter Twelve
A symphony of symptoms

9 times out of 10 when I see people who I
haven't seen for a while I can almost hear
their thoughts
– *'He doesn't look sick'* –
to be honest I am glad that the symptoms
aren't always purely physical because my God
if they were, they would terrify you.

I would like to write about the symptoms I was experiencing before some of my visits to see my neurologist. I kept a diary therefore you will see some dates are before and some are after I was diagnosed with LBD. As I have already mentioned I was diagnosed with LBD in May 2017.

April 2017 was a particularly bad time for me and I had kept a list of things that bothered me the most, so that I could let the neurologist know the details on subsequent visits.

1. Hip Pain

I seemed to have constant pain especially in my right hip and sometimes radiating across my back and into my left hip. As I had been diagnosed with Paget's disease in Australia having had a nuclear medical scan as I said earlier, they had told me that this disease was the cause of my hip pain, however, the specialist in Ireland following on from other scans believed that because the pain I had was so severe he didn't believe that Paget's was responsible. Two doctors, two countries and two different opinions. By this time, I was walking with the aid of a walking frame and it was around this time that I was put on Bu Trans patches of which the dosage was increased gradually, and I stayed on those until January 2018.

2. Blurred Vision

My sight seemed to be deteriorating a little when reading. I just got 1.5 reading glasses but now I was having a different problem in that I have blurred vision which is especially worse in the morning. It feels like there is a sheet of water in front of my eyes. This feeling can last up to a couple of hours and I still have it to this day. Not every day but especially after a night where I get very little sleep or if my head is just not feeling right. I don't know how to better describe it but there are times that my head just does not feel right and there are times I wonder is this it, is this when my brain finally gives up? I will at times write in the present tense and that is because I still have the same symptoms today.

3. Slurred speech

This is the first time that I noticed this and again to this day I can have this especially first thing in the morning. The best way to describe is it's like as if I am half drunk. I am sometimes aware of it and sometimes Helena might point it out to me saying *'you must be feeling bad this morning because I notice it in your voice'.* It sometimes feels very embarrassing especially if I am talking to someone who wouldn't have heard me slur my speech before. I do find however that my speech will return to normal within about fifteen minutes.

4. Handwriting

Now my handwriting was never very good, and I remember even at National School spending extra time trying to learn how to write properly. The best way for me to explain it to you is that I couldn't write a clear letter A, E or O. There would always be a line or part of a line through it. However, my handwriting could be read quite easily, and it was never a problem as far as exams or work was ever involved. Now this is different, as I write I go from big to small letters, very stretched out and from joined up writing to printing. I find that it takes extra concentration to write anything more than a few words and it has now gone to the stage where I can't even read my own writing after a couple of days. It is something that I have pretty much given up on and I need to keep a small diary with me at all times I now just write down words rather than sentences.

5. Sudden Sweating

Again, this still happens to me for no apparent reason. I just start to sweat so bad that my shirt gets wet and my forehead also, thankfully within a couple of minutes my temperature returns to normal. I suppose I could describe it as a car just overheating for a few minutes and then back to normal again. These episodes of sudden sweating don't happen with any great frequency nor can I say at any specific time. It happens just out of the blue maybe every day for five days and then may not happen again for a week or two, the only good thing about it is that it goes as quick as it comes.

6. Confusion

I have also noticed that my confusion is getting worse. I can now just be introduced to someone and within a couple of minutes I have forgotten the name. What's more disturbing for me is when family names are a problem for me. All too often nowadays I can get confused but when told the proper name I am OK. I can also get confused about what day, date or year it is.

7. Tremors

It presented itself at first in my left hand and right leg. I had noticed these tremors for a long time maybe even six months before I had ever gone to the neurologist. I am a 'Ciotog' which is a common Irish term used for a person who is left handed, therefore when this tremor developed in my left hand, at first I found it to be more of a nuisance than anything else. Then unfortunately it got worse, and it got so bad that I could not hold a glass or a cup because I would spill everything. Now I'm very glad to say that I have trained myself to use my right hand therefore I don't notice it as much anymore.

The amazing thing is that the tremor in my left hand does not seem to be as bad anymore now that the focus is off of it...I think! My right leg would just start to shake when I was lying down, I now know it's considered a resting tremor. I found it very noticeable if I was lying on the couch watching TV and this could continue for hours but now it has got to the stage where I really don't take much notice of it anymore, it doesn't bother me.

Sometimes I also have a tremor in my left leg but not as often as my right. The worst time for me is in the morning and especially if I have to get up within minutes of waking up. It's important for me to have at least 15mins sometimes longer as a transition period between waking and getting out of bed to get my bearings, almost like getting off a boat with the sea legs still intact. If when I wake up I just lay in bed for maybe fifteen minutes I can get out of bed as pretty normal. If I get out of bed within the first five minutes I will find it very hard to get my balance and there are times when it feels like my whole body is trembling and can be quite frightening because this feeling can last ten to fifteen minutes.

With this trembling comes slurred speech and you don't feel right. The thought sometimes enters my head... My God...what happens if this feeling doesn't stop. Is this it and if I'm not careful I could work myself into a bit of a panic attack quite easily. The best way I find to counteract it, is that I just try to ignore it and reassure myself that it will pass in a couple of minutes. I do believe that you can send the strongest message to your mind from yourself while being assertive about it.

'This will get better.....This too shall pass'

8. Stopping mid-sentence

Another symptom I sometimes have, and which really torments and embarrasses me is that I could be talking to you and suddenly stop mid- sentence and would have to ask what we were talking about. Thinking about this now I have to be honest and say that it has made me a little withdrawn in that not all the time but some of the time if I can get away without meeting people I will, because of it. Again, it's just another one of the tiny battles that I fight with, not on a daily basis but often enough. The thing about these little battles is that there is no telling when or where they are going to take place and that for me is the nasty bit and can at times be frightening.

9. Appetite

I always had a very good and healthy appetite, too good at times, but I have to say that since I left hospital in 2015 in Australia my appetite has never again been the same. Sometimes I can have such a big appetite, like I'm just starving with the hunger and no matter what I eat it's never enough or I can go for days and survive on just a small meal, there is no actual pattern to it. I have also found that when I feel hungry and while thinking of what I might eat I can go right off of the idea. This is especially obvious in the mornings. I would say to myself that I'd like to have a boiled egg and toast but by the time I get to the kitchen I find myself forcing down just a cup of tea. I try as best I can to have breakfast, dinner and supper but to be honest only succeed maybe two or three days a week. The rest is very mixed up, sometimes I might have one big meal before going to bed and some days I might have no proper meal.

10. Loud noise

Ever since I was a little boy I hated loud noises or sudden bangs - like for instance a car backfiring, it did then and still to this day it frightens me. But the biggest thing that I have noticed in the last two years, 2016 to now 2018 is that people talking loudly or crowds of people talking bother me. Something as simple as visitors calling and I have said to Helena on several occasions why is everyone shouting? There are even times when I will leave the room as I just cannot stand the loud noise. The same can be said of crowds, I will try as best I can to avoid places with crowds, especially family gatherings or where a lot of people want to talk to me.

I now find situations like that overwhelming, not all of the time but a lot of the time, again if possible I will avoid the situation. If someone even pops a piece of bubble-gum close to me it hurts my head but I have found lately that putting in my ear phones and listening to music is a great comfort to me. Funny thing is, the one thing I find worse than both loud noises or crowds is complete silence. When there is complete silence and calm, I can hear almost a constant buzzing in my brain. It is very faint but it's always there and that is as bad as any noise because I get the feeling that I am going mad and again it calls for me to be strong and to tell myself that I will be able to get out of the situation and fix it. It might be as simple as putting on the TV or radio in the background. For me nowadays complete silence is out of the question. Again, it's a question of finding a sort of happy medium.

11. Other symptoms

Diverticulitis

I had a colonoscopy done in 2016 which showed that I had diverticulitis which is a problem with the bowel and which I still have to this day. There are times when I get a flare up and when it does I feel pretty awful but then I can have a period when it settles down and all is OK.

Asthma

I was diagnosed with asthma in 2016 having spent a few days in hospital in Mallow with more chest pain. I also have sleep apnoea and I use the sleep apnoea machine whenever I sleep and find it very helpful, I will go into this in more detail later on.

Energy Levels

A few weeks ago my energy levels were at an all-time low, but I have to say that with a change in lifestyle, a daily routine and some light exercise they seem to be on the up again. Like everything in my life now, I have good days and bad days, but I'm beginning to see that the more structure I have in my day the better my energy levels seem to be.

As I mentioned at the beginning of the chapter these are pretty much the symptoms that I presented with on my second trip to see my neurologist in Cork.

Chapter Thirteen
They said it was impossible

Trying to not let my illness define me has been another hurdle to overcome, it really is a battle to take one day at a time and not let it consume me.

Helena and I had planned to visit our children and grandchildren in Sydney in late 2017, even though at this stage I had been diagnosed with Parkinson's Disease. Little did I know I had another hurdle before me as in May 2017 I was told that I had LBD.

All the family encouraged me to cancel my plans, but I was adamant I still wanted to go. At the time it seemed like a pipe dream, but the more I thought about it the more I wanted to do it. There seemed to be a lot of problems in the way but something inside me said that it was going to happen, and nothing was going to stop me.

There was the problem of the long journey, two big flights, seven hours to Dubai, and fourteen hours to Sydney and I used get so bored on the flights. How would I handle the flights now? What about travel insurance and what about my doctor? What would he say?

We went to my doctor and he seemed happy with the plan and gave me the go ahead to travel. As we lived 150 miles from Dublin we decided that we would travel to Dublin on a Monday morning, stay at a hotel near Dublin airport and fly out of Dublin on Tuesday evening at 5pm so that we would be flying at night. We had just a 7 hour flight to Dubai and as luck would have it, there is a beautiful hotel within the airport and we stayed there for 24 hours.

Instead of travelling the very long flight to Sydney we decided to fly to Perth which is about 5 hours shorter and my brother Tom, his wife Julie and their children live there. We were to spend a few days there, then it was a short flight to Melbourne to Helena's brother Dave and after a couple of days there it was just a short hop to Sydney to see our children and grandchildren and all our friends.

We booked our tickets and hotels and it was something wonderful to look forward to. It definitely kept me going and made me more determined than I had ever been to make this work. We stayed for seven weeks to allow lots of time for me to rest before the flight home again. It really gave me a focus and I made sure that I tried to keep myself and my mind as right as possible and sure enough before we knew it we were on our way and looking forward to seeing everyone. I carried quite a supply of medicine and at that time I was on a lot of it.

List of medication was as follows:

Bu Trans Patches 30mg

Co-Diovan 160/12.5

Amalode 10mg

Nexium 20 mg

Donesyn 10mg

Rivotril 10mg

SINEMET *There is a reason why I highlighted Sinemet and I will get to it shortly.*

My plan was as much as possible to keep taking my tablets as close to Irish time as possible and over a couple of days get into Australian time.

Just to go back a couple of months to July 1st when I was put on the Sinemet. I started on a small dose and over the space of a month gradually increased it up to the dose I was to continue on and that went OK, until the day that I reached the top dose and within a matter of hours I got violently sick. I was vomiting and I had a fever one minute and was freezing the next and back again to burning up. That happened on a Sunday and we were staying 45 miles from home. After a terrible night, on the Monday morning we got into the car and went straight to my doctor, I was only able to stand up with the help of Helena as I felt so ill.

I am lucky enough to have a wonderful GP and as soon as he examined me he sent me straight to hospital in Mallow where I would spend the next nine days in isolation, as I was so ill they couldn't take the chance of putting me in a ward with other people. Visitors were limited to close family and they had to wear masks and gloves when visiting me. They wondered if it may have been a reaction to the Sinemet but because I had so many different complications it was difficult to pin down the cause. I was started back on the Sinemet again but on a much smaller dose and this was gradually raised over a longer period of time and it seemed to be going OK even though every now and then I would feel a little nauseous.

Now back to Australia, everything was going to plan, the hotels beautiful, flights lovely and it wasn't long before I was reunited with my brother Tom at the airport in Perth. Tom and I have always been very close and he along with his wife Julie, since the day I was first diagnosed with the Parkinson's Disease have been such support and literally a pillar of strength for me. We speak at least once a week, even though I am older he has really taken over as my big brother.

On my second evening in Perth I was not feeling the best and even though we were supposed to go out for the night I said that I wasn't feeling right and would go to bed early at around 7pm, I was putting it down to jetlag and thought a good night's sleep would work.

I went to bed and was sleeping on and off until about 4am when I awoke, and I knew that something was very wrong again. I called Tom and himself and Julie came into the room, luckily for me Julie is a nurse and she took one look at me and knew that I was in trouble.

Over the course of the next couple of hours I was starting to burn up again and she knew exactly what to do. She contacted a doctor where she worked and between them they finally got my temperature down and stopped the vomiting. At one stage she mentioned that maybe it was time to call an ambulance. Julie drew on all her nursing skills and got me through it and a decision was made for me to once again stop taking the Sinemet. After about four days I was good enough to fly to

Sydney and the rest of the trip went pretty much without incident even though there were days when I was not feeling great. On good days I would enjoy myself and on bad days I would just relax and take care of myself. It's a very good idea to know your limits.

I have to thank my brother Tom, Julie their wonderful Children Mick, Sarah, Tom Junior who is my Godson and Rob for the wonderful care they showed me, and I have to apologise for giving them a fright. Even their dog tried to comfort me by putting his paw on me every time I would lie down. I must say that I'm delighted with myself for making that trip and we had a fantastic holiday with the Children and especially great fun with the grandchildren Charlie and Liam.

Chapter Fourteen
Lewy Body is taking over

I know that to some people a person living with dementia may be challenging to deal with, giving others a hard time but the sad reality is that a person living with dementia is having a hard time.

I went to the outpatients' department in the hospital to meet with my neurologist early January 2018. This was a regular appointment as part of my usual check-ups. For eleven days leading up to this I had not slept for eleven nights in a row and when I say I didn't sleep, I would go to bed exhausted, my balance was so bad with sheer exhaustion that I had to hold onto something or I would fall. As soon as my head would hit the pillow I knew that it was no use, no way could I fall asleep. It was like my brain simply would not shut down for the night no matter how I twisted or turned, no good.

I tried to sleep with the Sleep Apnoea machine on but no good, with the mask off no good. I would get up again and lie down on the couch, turn on the TV but was too agitated to watch anything, feeling exhausted I would go back to bed again. Same thing the thoughts going through your mind were, My God I cannot go on like this night after night maybe I would be better off to end my life right now. At this point I can tell you is that this is probably the loneliest place to be feeling depressed, agitated, angry, helpless, alone while also being filled with rage on a couple of occasions that I was letting it get the better of me and I could see that it was getting to me.

Then through sheer exhaustion I might nod off to sleep for instance at 5am, only to wake again ten minutes later and this torment went on day and night for as I said eleven days before I visited my neurosurgeon. I must have looked pretty bad when we went into her because after talking to me for five minutes she would need to do some further tests and would like to admit me to hospital there and then. She told me that one of the benefits of being admitted would be that I could see a consultant psychiatrist who she recommended. I have to say at this stage, that my neurologist has been brilliant to me since my very first appointment, therefore I knew whatever she recommended would be in my best interest.

I was admitted on Wednesday evening and would remain in hospital in the acute stroke ward until the following Tuesday. I met with the new consultant who took me off of the antidepressant medication that I was taking, and he also took me off of the Bu Trans 30mg pain patches and this was done in increments of 5mg over the next few weeks. The dose of

Rivotril and Donesyn were increased in order to help me sleep better and for the first couple of nights thankfully the sleep started to improve. As usual in the hospital my medication was monitored and with the changes I started to get a few hours' sleep.

The only problem was when I would wake up in the middle of the night, I didn't have a clue where I was, who I was or what was happening. It was very frightening. On one of the nights when I woke up, I drool a lot in my sleep whether I am wearing the sleep apnoea mask or not, but I thought that my face was dripping blood. I could feel it, but I couldn't see it and in my confused state I wandered out to the hallway. A lovely nurse helped me back to bed and spent time reassuring me that everything was all right. I am so thankful for her kindness and patience.

When I wake at night, there are times I feel like a lost and lonely child and need the very same reassurance that you would give a young child or even a baby. That lovely nurse, spoke to me in a very soft and caring voice which for me as a LBD patient is so very important. Little things like it's going to be OK, are you OK, telling me where I am and answering my questions honestly was and is so important to me.

It is the same at home when I wake at night when I look at Helena, I may not even recognise her face but when she speaks then I recognise her voice and it makes all the difference. Again, she reassures me that everything is all right and also that I am safe and at home.

The consultant psychiatrist over a period of a few days went over my complete medical history in pretty good detail from start to finish and went through all of my hospital visits in Ireland as well as from Australia. Then on the Monday evening he asked me if Helena could come in on the Tuesday morning as he wanted to meet both of us together and all going well I could go home. We both met with the consultant on the Tuesday morning and he explained that there was nothing that could be done for my Lewy Body Dementia, but they could help me with the nightmares, the confusion and hopefully the sleep or to be more precise my complete lack of sleep.

I asked him directly. How long had I left before I actually lost my mind or before the LBD took over completely? ....and his answer was that he could not say as every patient is different.

As I am one of those patients who prefers to know all the facts, because when I do I feel hopeful that I can do something about the problem whatever it is or however big or small it is. I was not as shocked as you might think to be told that there was no more they could really do for me as I half expected it from what research I had done on LBD, but I was delighted at what he did tell me.

He told me:

1. I did not have a mental illness

2. I did not suffer from depression

Right there and then I knew that I had a fighting chance against suicide, having read all about the actor Robin Williams and of his sad passing by taking his own life.

His wife Susan had said that Robin was on anti- depressant medication and the autopsy after his death confirmed that he also had LBD. Knowing how low and down I can feel because of it, I couldn't help thinking that if on top of LBD, I also suffered from depression which in my estimation would mean that I had no chance at all.

When I was told that I did not suffer from depression I was so relieved. I felt immediately that the chances of dying at the hands of suicide had greatly reduced. I actually left the hospital in a better and balanced frame of mind and as the saying goes...'grateful for little mercies'.

Chapter Fifteen
An ugly disease

Nothing prepares you for this disease. No one is prepared for the isolation, friends disappear because the person they knew is no longer there. The caregiver gets trapped with the patient. It is very lonely and isolating.

Meryl Comer

This trip to hospital has taught me a very valuable lesson that when a person suffers from LBD it is of enormous importance that the difference between suffering from depression and the symptoms of LBD are not mixed up.

It is definitely true to say that a lot of them can be similar, it is of vital importance that you sit down and talk to the proper professional to determine which is which. Do I get sad and very lonely at times, of course I do I am suffering from an incurable disease and I remember one doctor calling it 'this ugly disease' and by God he was right. The way I try and bring myself out of it is to think of the positive things in my life. My wife, my children, my grandchildren, my wonderful friends and family and I make sure that I have always something to look forward to.

Do I feel suicidal at times unfortunately the answer is the very same, of course I do but more importantly the solution is the same. Without doubt and I cannot stress this enough talk to someone that you trust, write it down if you can and if you are on your own even record your feelings into your phone if you have to but do not under any circumstances bottle things up.

For me, the more I tell my wife Helena what exactly is going on in my head the better my head is for cleaning out all the rubbish in there. I am not saying that the thoughts and feelings go away the very minute that I talk about them, but it really helps. Another thing I do, and this was at the suggestion of the doctor is I now have structure in my day and I have found this to be very helpful. Before this trip to hospital I got up if I wasn't too tired but if I was very tired I stayed in bed. I will give you an example of a typical day for me now and this is almost twelve months on from being diagnosed with LBD.

I try to get up at around 8am and have a cup of tea and toast and take my tablets, I take two tablespoons of hemp oil and some CBD oil as it has helped with my tremor and my pain. I will look at my phone, check some emails, check in with some friends and also speak on social media with people from around the world who are suffering from the same horrific disease as me. I will go to the room and sit or lie down and meditate using the headspace app or I may choose to listen to one of the other meditation apps that I have. That five to ten minutes that I spend on meditation helps me to check in to see exactly what way I am feeling and also to confirm what kind of a mood I am in. This allows me to fix it if I want to sometimes I do, sometimes I don't.

Then depending on the weather, I will do some light gardening or some few jobs in my little workshop. I will also take time out most mornings to do some writing. Other days I will go for a drive with my good friend Flor who has been there for me as a friend for a lifetime. We chat and laugh about the good old days and our lives now. Don't ever underestimate the value of a good friend. I try not go to bed in the afternoons anymore unless I'm very tired but you most of the time I don't sleep anyway.

I find it is of vital importance to have something to look forward to like a trip or a holiday or a visitor calling but find that something you want to do and plan for it. Do not put off a trip unless you have to, everyone said that I wouldn't be able for the trip to

Australia in October 2017 but I went for seven weeks, had some bad days but mainly good.

Plan your life and live it to the full, don't stop planning because of Lewy Body Dementia.

I try as best I can to eat breakfast lunch and supper and once a week at least I go to the local pub for a few drinks to meet the locals, sometimes I have to push myself and that is good too, I don't push myself too hard but sometimes I have to in order to get out and meet different people. Another thing that I find very helpful is jigsaws. Start off small and work up. The bottom line is I try to keep my brain as active as I possibly can for as long as I can each and every day.

Some days it doesn't work but by in large it is working for me.

Another very important thing for me is if I say that I want to be left alone then that is what I want, and I think it should apply to most LBD sufferers when asking them what they want. Please be prepared to do as they ask providing it is safe to do so obviously. It's OK to check in with them. I find for myself that my granddaughter Hollie who is now 8 years old has a great way of asking and listening.

Children are brilliant at that because they are talking to the person who they know and love and not the disease.

Chapter Sixteen

REM sleep behaviour disorder

I have had to try and let go of worrying, to enjoy the now and not worry too much about tomorrow – easier said than done!

For a couple of months each time I went into a dream, it would very quickly turn into a nightmare. Subsequently my Neurologist diagnosed me with REM Sleep Behaviour Disorder...RBD.

I would often wake in the mornings and tell Helena that my dreams were so real that it seemed like I was living in a completely different world. My dreams were so real and so detailed that it would take me a couple of minutes to figure out where I was when I would wake in the morning.

Now I use the word dreams lightly. They were and still are nightmares and the longer I have LBD the worse they are getting. As each night passes the amount and quality of sleep I am getting is less and less, some nights I might only get three hours sleep and as a result my wife doesn't get a quality nights' sleep either. I will give you just a few examples of the nightmares. I could not write all of the details as they are very frightening.

One night I was dreaming that I was living in America in an apartment block and while in a public toilet I could see these two teenagers with what seemed like a quilt from a bed and they were cutting it up in strips. I didn't want to say anything to them as I felt it was a bad area and as they had a knife I didn't feel safe. I went outside and was talking to my Uncle Dave who had died from Alzheimer's Disease in real life.

When I went back in, one of the teenagers was hanging and had used the strips they had cut from the quilt. I called the police and was unable to tell them the address therefore I was in a panic. I gave the phone to a woman and told her to give the policeman on the other end all the details. Reading this you will have noticed, I am only relating half the story but I could not add all the other horrific things that happened. I just wanted to give you a glimpse of the vivid nightmares I experience all too often.

Then I awoke absolutely petrified. I took of my sleep apnoea mask as I was so thirsty and needed to go to the bathroom but was frozen in fear. As usual Helena obviously helped me through this episode and for the next two and half hours, I lay in bed reliving the nightmare and terrified that someone would walk down the hall and into the bedroom. For me this is very common at night, I fear that someone will

For some reason I was involved in murdering a man and had the body buried in a ditch, but the murder had taken place a good few months back. Every night I could feel the worry, what if the body was ever discovered, I could wind up in jail, what would my friends think of me especially as one of my friends is a policeman. I have no idea who was murdered or why, but it was again terrifying to be living in this nightmare, the worry and stress of it all. It was so real, and I decided to move the body to where I do not know. All I remember was the horrible smell, I suddenly woke out of the nightmare but one thing that didn't leave me all the following day was the smell. It was so bad that Helena decided to go to the health shop and she bought some orange essential oil. I put some under my nostrils to try to get rid of the smell and it helped a little.

The frightening thing about these nightmares is walking up from them, not being able to go back to sleep and in most cases afraid of going back to sleep just in case I would go back into the same dream again, which often happens. There are days when all that I can think about are the nightmares from the night before and I can get so caught up in them that before I know it my day has gone, and the cycle starts all over again.

I can honestly say at this stage that the worst part of the LBD for me at the moment are the nights and the REM Sleep Behaviour Disorder. It has happened me on a few occasions where I have woken up from another terrifying nightmare looked at my wife Helena who would be asleep beside me and shouted at her...... who are you?.... it is only when she spoke that I realised it was Helena and again she has the job of comforting me and telling me that everything is OK and that I am at home safe and sound in my own bed.

I suppose every disease affects those who are closest to you but I can say none more so than LBD, because my wife has as many sleepless nights as I do and when she sleeps I don't think she even gets a proper sleep because she is so conscious of what I am going through and at times probably worried that I might attack her by acting out one of my dreams.

I could write books about the different dreams but there is no point, none of them are about lying on a beach somewhere sipping a cocktail, instead they are all about murder, death and mayhem.

That would be my worst nightmare to do anything to hurt my wife and it is something that we have had to discuss, and if the day comes that she thinks that she is in any danger whatsoever, then we will have separate bedrooms. We have discussed a dementia facility for when my disease progresses. It is so important to discuss all these issues with your loved ones especially when your mind is still pretty good.

At the end of the book I will give a list of practical steps that we took should the day come that I can no longer think or do things for myself.

Chapter Seventeen
My tips on living with LBD

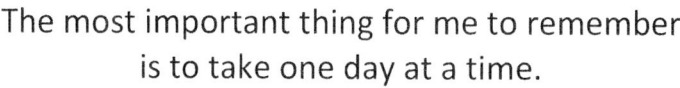

The most important thing for me to remember
is to take one day at a time.

There are a lot of things that can be done to help a person and indeed the family of someone who is suffering from this horrible disease.

Of course, it depends on each persons' different circumstances, but I will tell you what helps me and especially Helena who is actually on the front line of this every day.

Recognise the person and not the disease.

- **You are not your illness**
- **You have a name, a history and a personality**
- **Staying yourself is an on - going battle**

I am Kevin, I am a Husband, I am a Father, I am a Grandfather, I am a Godfather, I am a Son, I am a Brother and I am a Friend and I also have Lewy Body Dementia. I put things in that order for a reason and that is because sometimes when people look at others with dementia, all they might see is the disease and not who the person really is.

One great example of this is the way my Grandchildren look at me when they see me they see me as their Grandfather and not a person with a disease, now they do know what is wrong with me, but they can look past that and see the person and luckily they seem to have a great understanding of me.

I mentioned earlier the book 'Feathers in my Brain' by the Crystal Project in Ireland and both my eldest Granddaughter Hollie and myself read it together, it is a beautifully illustrated book and gently explains Dementia to children.

Although it was a little sad to hear her reading it aloud, we also had fun when we acted out some of the pictures.

Remember that the person with dementia is changing and I know for sure that I am changing.

Don't tell someone get over it

Help them to get through it

For me there have been a lot of changes within myself and with my thinking. One example is my mood, it can change from day to day and sometimes from hour to hour. I find that sometimes I can be very quick tempered especially with Helena, (they say you hurt the ones you love the most). I can fly off the handle very fast, shout and demand that I am left alone, thankfully not very often, but it has happened.

I do not want to try to minimise it because sometimes I can see the pain and the hurt in her eyes and that is not right.

Just something as simple as asking if I would like a cup of tea and I say no, but then she may ask again or say are you sure? *I am thinking in my mind what part of no do you not understand.*

I have found that talking openly about things like this is the best policy and now Helena asks me once and if the answer is no, then she leaves it at that. Also, if there is something that we don't agree on, we leave it alone and usually return to it a short time later and it's usually resolved. This approach has worked very well for me and I feel that it lessons my frustration.

Getting Physically Violent

The one thing that terrifies me is that I have been asked by more than one of my medical team if I have ever shown violence towards my wife and up to the time of writing, thank God I haven't been and hope I never will.

However, with LBD it's very possible that it might happen or may even occur in my sleep if I start acting out one of my nightmares. We have discussed it at length and if at any point it looks like it might happen, then I will have no choice but to leave our bedroom and sleep in another room.

If it happens while I am awake and conscious, well then that's another story on another level altogether. God forbid, if I get to the point that I am violent I have made it quite clear that I will need to be admitted to a facility for people with dementia. I can still have lots of visitors and have days out as often as I would like, but for me it's just not right that the person living with me should be living in fear of being hit or attacked. It was very important for me to have this conversation with Helena while my mind is still in good order.

It is now twelve months since I have been diagnosed with LBD and my mind is still in good condition therefore now is the time to have these important conversations.

You cannot be strong all the time

Sometimes you just need to be left alone

To let the tears out

Power of Attorney

Another thing that we did was go to see our solicitor to make sure that our wills are up to date and we also discussed putting in place the power of attorney.

That simply means, when my wife can see that I'm no longer capable of making decisions for myself, the doctor will then go to court with my solicitor and appointed family members to fulfil my wishes.

It involves my wife, children, one of my brothers, my doctor and my solicitor and above all it has given both myself and Helena a bit of peace of mind knowing that when the day comes, and intervention is needed, all will be well in the knowledge that my plan was hatched when my mind was still active.

Parties and Family Gatherings

I was a very sociable person and loved nothing more than a good party.

Shortly before I was diagnosed with Parkinson's Disease I was actually a DJ and used to mime to the music and loved nothing better than a good night out. In the last twelve months I am actually afraid to be out late at night, hate being in large crowds or being in a place that is very noisy or has loud music. It is not that I love peace and quiet because as I mentioned earlier in the book, that brings with it a host of other problems. It is that I just can't tolerate loud noise as it hurts my brain, therefore I do not put pressure on myself to go, nowadays not even to family events.

There are times when family members don't understand dementia but maybe they are just afraid of it or may just simply be in denial of it. I have gone to a few parties but felt so uncomfortable and felt so unsafe in myself, that I left within an hour of getting there. I have been to two weddings where I've had to leave after the meal. Now if we go to a family wedding we book a room in the hotel where I can go to bed if I don't feel comfortable and Helena can still enjoy herself, knowing that I'm safe and sound.

There are days also that I will just not feel well enough to go and will choose to stay at home.

TIP: If I am ever invited to anything now, I tell them that I have LBD and to expect me if they see me and at this stage it is very comforting to know that if I don't turn up they will more than understand.

I try to get out at least once a week during the day for a few drinks, have a laugh with some others and I must say that I think it's actually beneficial for the body, mind and spirit. They know about my condition, treat me as normal and even though there are days that I don't feel like going I try and make myself get up and get on with it.

I know it's good to get out and meet the people, maybe even just talk about sport or conversations to right all wrongs, but at least it's a different focus.

Being honest with my family

My beautiful daughter Noreen who lives in Australia got engaged recently and is planning to get married in Australia in two years' time. Being the proud daddy, I must say that I have always looked forward to giving my daughter away on her wedding day but it has always been her wish to get married in Australia and unfortunately it is possible, depending on the progression of my LBD, that I may be unable to be at her side on her special day, I feel sad at the thought of it.

I have discussed this at length with Noreen and while she was then going to change her plans I was insistent that she would do no such thing. I have told her that if my head is right I will be there on the day and if my head is not - then I won't.

My point here is that if my head is not right then it does not matter because I will not remember it and I will not have to be looked after on her day. She will come home afterwards, and we can get photos then, but I do believe it is pointless to destroy her plans because of Lewy Body Dementia. It's my way of not letting it win or not letting it ruin my daughter's big day.

Funeral

None of us know how much time
We have left on this earth
What is left in the end are your memories
Your actions and how people felt about you
So, try and leave behind
Memories of love and good times

Nobody knows when they are going to die but we all will someday.

As the diagnoses of LBD is a sick one in every sense of the word and the life span might not be very long. This fact has led to many discussions that I've had with Helena and the children and I have told them what I would like, and they have told me the same.

I find that by having all of these little chats, it has brought a lot of peace of mind to all of us and we are not denying the reality of the situation, nor are we putting off difficult decisions. If something should happen suddenly to me, those who I love and are dear to me know exactly what my wishes are.

Something that really surprised me was that I had always wanted to be cremated but when I said that to my children they got quite upset and said that they couldn't stand the idea of it. On the other hand, I never liked the thought of being buried.

It was a topic that we left alone for a while, until one day the answer came to me. I decided to donate my body to science as they might be able to understand the cause of some if not all of my other ailments and also might provide a window into this horrible disease. The real bonus is that my children are happy with my decision also. The thought of been buried two years after dying is not as frightening to me.

Reality

Reality to someone suffering from dementia and reality for people who don't can often be very different and that's OK.
Don't ever dismiss what we are saying, for example if I say that there is a cat in the room don't say that there isn't or dismiss it, instead ask about it what kind is it, ask do I like cats, ask did I ever have a cat, it just might bring back some lovely memories to me and be the start of a lovely conversation.

On the other hand, if I hate cats say that you will hunt out the cat and ask if the cat is gone, it just might make a big difference and bring comfort to me in my reality.

I believe that it is important to listen to every request and if possible, safe and reasonable to do so, what is the harm in doing it. Sometimes I might be in the middle of a sentence and for no reason other than LBD I can stop mid-sentence and forget what I was saying. My advice here is just to wait for a couple of seconds and if I don't remember what I was saying just gently remind me. I think one of the worst things that can be done is that what we are saying is dismissed or shrugged off, it is a small thing that will bring back a memory.

I recently visited the beautiful Care Bright Dementia Village in Bruff in County Limerick in Ireland and visited with some of the service users living there. I spoke with two women and while they did not know how long they had been residents, and one of them had to be told where she was from, when I mentioned people that I knew from where they lived they remembered and we were able to have a conversation about the different families and I could see that it brought a smile to their faces. They could again interact.

**When a person with dementia says
I want to go home
Home is often a feeling
Rather than a physical place**

Stigma

I have found that in some places and in some families, there is still a stigma attached to dementia with almost a cloak of silence thrown over it.

That is so wrong, and we must all work towards eliminating it. As far as I'm concerned, I have a disease like any other but with devastating consequences and I have no problem whatsoever telling everyone I meet and sharing with them how bad my days can be from time to time. This helps me and also helps to explain to the other person why I am the way I am, and I also believe that sharing how I feel to others will help to dissolve the ignorance around dementia somewhat.

**We live in a world where if you break your leg
Everyone wants to sign your cast
But if you tell people that you have dementia**

Some people run the other way
To some people
Any part of your body can break down
Except for your mind

Education

Nowadays there is so much educational material on dementia and organisations together with some brilliant social media groups from all over the world that people can join. So much information about what works and what doesn't work for different people and the way dementia is dealt with in different countries. I find that when people share their experiences it can be very helpful, but I would never do anything without first discussing it with my doctor or indeed never ever change medication without your doctor's advice.

Hobbies and Pastimes

For me it is of vital importance to have some hobbies and pastimes because there are times when I might not go outside for two or three days at a time and it is so important to have something to do. One thing that I find to be particularly hard to deal with is cold and wet weather. So, when the weather is getting better and at the very least dry I love to do a bit of gardening and even though I am not able to do a lot of digging there are machines and family who are only too willing to help. I love planting and this year I hope to have a nice vegetable garden.

I also have a small little workshop where I cut up timber for the fire and every now and then make little things like flower boxes. It my 'man cave' where I also I keep things in jam jars like screws and nails and of course my tools and my ride on lawnmower which I love to use. I love to be outside and as we live in the countryside I love the fresh air and the sound of the birds singing. They might sound like small things, but it gives me great pleasure and again peace of mind. The reason I use this term 'peace of mind' so often is because with LBD, a lot of the time I can assure you that it is very hard to come by.

As I have said earlier, the quiet of the dead of night really does my head in, while in contrast the noise from the birds and a light breeze on a nice day is just so relaxing. While I am in the garden there is always a little robin there and for me it really is a wonderful place to be. If my mind is not feeling right it is a great place to go for peace and tranquillity. I also try to keep a couple of hens and find them very therapeutic as they seem to have their own individual personalities and that is also good for my mind as well as their fresh organic eggs.

I sometimes spend a day collecting cattle with my friend Flor who is a farmer and cattle dealer. These very enjoyable days, takes me out of the house, gives Helena a well-deserved break from me, while also having the added bonus of time to chat about what's going on with me and it feels good at times to have someone else to talk to. I love horseracing and have a couple of other great friends who enjoy racing as much as I do, and when I am able they will take me racing for a day.

Family support is all important, but I cannot stress enough the importance of friends also, and I think it has a lot to do with the fact that you don't meet them every day but when you do it is something new and fresh and again. It's very good for my mind.

I love watching sport and again I find it takes me away from my mind. I do not go to as many games as I used to or would like to because of the crowds but I do try to watch a lot of sport on TV and again I find it beneficial for my mind and it was something that was always part of my life.

Driving

I have found talking to different people that this is a very difficult with some dementia sufferers. If you are used to driving yourself everywhere or if you're the spouse that always took the wheel on the Sunday drive, then if that is suddenly taken away it can ignite within you a terrible feeling of loss. All of a sudden you have been driving all of your life and then one day that is gone, your independence is gone, and you are now depending on someone else to be your taxi service.

I have found it very challenging and I will tell you how Helena and I dealt with it. When I was diagnosed with Parkinson's Disease we started talking about it and we realized that the time would come when it was going to happen. We live about three miles from the nearest town and when we would go there together it was natural for me to be in the driver's seat.

Slowly but surely, I started taking the back seat as it were therefore for us it was an easy transition as I always felt that if I really needed to I could and I was still insured to drive so I felt it was a choice, it was not that I couldn't drive, it was that I chose not to drive.

Approximately twelve months after being diagnosed with Parkinson's Disease I was diagnosed with LBD. That day I made up my mind never to drive again, this was not a choice anymore as I knew there and then that I had to make this decision for me, my family and all other road users.

With Helena's help and more tears to wash away the shock of it all. I suppose it's like giving up anything there is always going to be a 'bit of cold turkey' and also taking away some freedom from both of us. Now if I need to go someplace and Helena doesn't, then it means that both of us have to go. I loved driving and some days I miss it terribly especially the freedom it gave me, even just going for a drive on my own listening to a tape of Joe Dolan, I was in a world of my own.

I didn't want to wait for a doctor to tell me that I could no longer drive but when I did tell my GP he thought that it was a very good idea. In a way I still felt it was my decision as nobody told me to stop driving and it was not because of this horrible disease, well in my mind anyway.

Again, it was a decision that I needed to make before my mind started to go, but above all one of the biggest factors was that if I was involved in an accident and people got hurt or killed and it was my fault. *'How could I live with myself'* and if the insurance company found out that I was driving with Lewy Body Dementia the chances are that I would not have been insured at all, maybe with some horrific consequences. *'That is not right, not right to visit my problems on other innocent people.'*

It has got a lot easier now that I am not driving but there are days when I still miss it and there are days that I tell Helena that she is not driving properly, but on the upside, I know that Helena is actually a great driver.

It is a discussion that you need to have with your loved one and my advice is the earlier the better. As it has turned out, for me it was the correct decision because on a couple of occasions I have seen cars coming towards us when in fact there has not been a car there. On a few occasions I have shouted at Helena to watch that person walking when there was evidently nobody there.

I do have hallucinations every now and then but take the following tablets for it:

DONEPEZIL HYDROCHLORIDE 10MG

I take them at night and find they have helped the hallucinations.

Talking in front of me

I like to call this *'Talking behind my back ....in front of me'*.
What I mean by this is that if Helena and I are out together or indeed if someone calls to visit. While I am in their company and within earshot they might actually say to Helena in front of me....'how is he today, he seems fine'.... as if I'm invisible. Now if you knew me, you would know that I am a big man and it would be pretty difficult for me to become invisible.

Please don't do that.... I am not deaf or invisible I have Lewy Body Dementia, instead ask me how I am doing today, ask me how I am feeling, you'd never know I might be just able to answer for myself and if I am not sure I can then bring Helena into the conversation by saying that I was good yesterday wasn't I or I had a bad day or whatever.

It does not matter what the conversation is, please don't dismiss the person with dementia and please listen to what they have to say and while you are listening, make sure you hear.

How I am today

This book has been on the go for the past nine months, and has been a lot of work. I can honestly say that when I started it I never thought that I would finish it but thankfully I have.

I want to let you know how I feel today now that the book is finished, approximately fifteen months after being diagnosed with Lewy Body Dementia. It really is a horrible disease.

I can feel LBD progressing in me but slowly and I'm finally beginning to accept this diagnosis and feel maybe acceptance is good. I have recently started to see my councillor PJ O Neill in Tralee again, because there are days when it all becomes a little overwhelming and I believe he has a good understanding of me and how my mind works.

I have become involved in a dementia working group in Ireland and it is so wonderful to meet people in the same situation as myself and to see what help is out there for all of us dementia sufferers. I found it very difficult to accept that even though I can stay at home alone for short periods during the day, I can no longer live alone. This reality was very painful and difficult to accept.

My nights are a little better than they used to be, in that I seem to be getting more sleep but I still have to deal with very upsetting dreams. The nightmares are as frightening and as violent as ever but I feel these are not happening with the same frequency as they used to. I find it helpful to listen to sleep meditation.

I got a bad urinary tract infection a couple of weeks ago and didn't say anything about it for two days. That was a bad mistake as the doctor had to be called late at night, such was the pain. I was put on a course of antibiotics for seven days, but would have saved Helena the stress of it all, saved the doctor a trip to the house and saved myself a lot of pain, if only I had spoken up earlier. Lesson learnt!

Lately I have found my anger and agitation levels raised and my tolerance level in general decreased. Some days I am well aware that my memory is fading a little and find it very frustrating. I sometimes struggle to remember what happened yesterday or which day of the week it is.

My energy levels can be extremely low at times and some days I am just unable to do anything but on a good day I love to get out to do some gardening. It is important for me to be aware of my limitations and to take longer breaks than I used to. Sometimes I can get carried away to another world while in my garden and I love it.

I really hope this book has helped you or a loved one who may be wrestling with LBD.

If you would like to contact me, my email is as follows: **kevinquaid9@gmail.com**

I would love to hear your comments and my plan is to follow up this book with personal YouTube videos on a regular basis.

My friends……don't ever give up the fight and never let Lewy Body Dementia win!

CHAPTER EIGHTEEN

Family & friends

It's terrifying for the patient

It's terrifying for the family

It's terrifying for the friends

But together- we will get through it

I have written a lot about the importance of family and friends in my life, therefore I asked some of my family and friends to put on paper what their thoughts are with regards to my diagnosis of Lewy Body Dementia.

Reading their thoughts unleashed within me a tsunami of tears and even though these thoughts are very personal to Me.......

I'm hopeful that they will also help you, especially if you or a loved one have been diagnosed with this disease.

Noreen Quaid

My eldest & Daddy's little girl

I have a favourite quote from Dr Seuss and it reads: **'Sometimes you will never know the value of a moment until it becomes a memory'**

That quote has always left such an impression on me, I think I was about 15 when I first came across it – little did I think the significant change in meaning it would have for me 15 years later.

Finding out my Dad had Lewy Body Dementia was a tough thought to process. My Dad – such a big and powerful man in every sense of the word, was all of a sudden given this diagnosis, something he nor I could control. That was not an easy thing to process but we are slowly getting our heads around it.

Memories are what make up a life, they give you comfort when you are down, fill you with love when you reminisce and remind you to be strong when times are tough. As the quote *says* **'you never know the value of a moment until it becomes a memory'.**

While they are precious they will not define my Dad, nor will I allow them to – he may lose some memories or struggle to recall but I will always be there to remind him of our moments – to reinforce their value, to ensure he knows he's loved – always has and always will be

Love you lots Dad

Noreen

Pat Quaid

Son

To be asked to give my thoughts and feelings on how my Dad's illness has impacted on my life is both a privilege and deeply saddening. Growing up with my Dad was like growing up with my own Superhero. For me this is how best to describe how I see and feel about my Father.

We have always been extremely close and when I was told that Dad had developed Lewy Body Dementia it was a huge shock as my Dad has always been the life of the party, the hard worker, the one who always bounced back. It's very hard to watch my Dad's health deteriorate, his day to day living and his many lifestyle changes.

My advice to anybody reading this in my Dad's book, is to cherish the moments you have together and think positively about the situation even though this may be difficult at times to do.

For me, I look at my Dad's illness Lewy Body Dementia as almost a lottery. What were the chances? Why my Dad? Why my Superhero?

I unfortunately ask myself these questions on a daily basis and have yet to find the answer!

I will finish with:

Love your family for their faults and fortunes, wrongs and rights and be there for them in their time of need.

Love you Dad, you will always be my Superhero, no matter what.

Paddy

Kevin Quaid Jnr

Son

When I was told my Father had been diagnosed with Parkinson's Disease, it was not very easy to accept but to add Lewy Body Dementia on top of it, was just impossible to accept even though he had been sick for a long time at this stage with lots of hospital visits.

I always thought of my Dad as youthful, full of fun and always up for anything. He loved socialising with my friends and they loved listening to him as he recalled his exploits as a young fella growing up in Co Limerick.

When we went surfing together in Sydney, well in Dad's case not really surfing but actually lying on the surf board on top of the waves trying to look good. He would be so proud if he caught a wave and I would hear all about it for days on end.

Sadly that is no longer the case as his energetic days are now few and far between. When I call to Dad and Helena these days, there is always the chance that he may be in bed, feeling unwell or just tired and lethargic.

My Dad, a big strong man in his early 50's. My Dad who loved the outdoors and lived life to the full. My Dad who was constantly on the move being told 'you have an incurable disease' and still trying to stay as positive as possible in the midst of it all....is truly inspiring.

With the help and support of his family and friends we will always be there for him. I didn't know anything about this frightful disease until Dad was diagnosed and I can now see that living with Lewy Body Disease on a daily basis is a very tough road to travel and on a bad day, I can see the pain and suffering on his face.

I will never give up on you Dad no matter what the future holds just as you never gave up on me.

Thank you Dad.

Kevin Quaid Jnr

Declan O'Connell

Stepson

For as long as I have known Kevin, my Stepdad he has always been very fit and active, whether it was playing golf, getting fit for his adventurous trip to Peru or working long hours in construction. When I worked with him in Australia he was always an early riser and prided himself on being fitter than most who were half his age.

All was well until Kevin started having health issues followed by numerous hospital admissions. It was plain to see that each hospital admission was taking its' toll and his recovery was taking longer each time which eventually made it impossible for him to work in construction any longer.

Mom and Kevin returned home to Ireland due to Kevin's ill health and in the past few years he still had to contend with more trips to hospital and many more health issues that seemed to be never ending. When we met up again a few months ago, the physical changes in Kevin were obvious. I was saddened to see that he looked older than his years and walked with the aid of a walking stick and lots of pain relieving medication. Mentally he was great, full of fun and still up for a joke and a laugh as he had always been, but the strong hard-working construction guy wasn't there anymore.

I could clearly see that physically this destructive disease called Lewy Body Dementia had progressed very quickly and I hope the dementia side of this disease progresses at a much slower rate as I have plans to have a lot more good times with you Kev.

Declan

Shane O'Connell

Stepson

Kevin has been my Stepdad for almost 20 years although I have known him for over 25. The following is Kevin's journey from my point of view.

I said goodbye to my Mother and my very healthy Stepfather in 2007 and emigrated to Australia. 18 months later both Mom and Kevin arrived in Sydney for my wedding and loved the place, driven by Kevin's sense of adventure they almost immediately started to plan their own adventure….. 'A five-year plan to live and work in Australia'.

Little did I know the Kevin that arrived in Australia full of life would not be the Kevin I would say goodbye to in a hospital bed 5 years later. It all started out great, I had been surrounded by my family and we would get together almost every weekend to enjoy nights' out, barbeques, football matches etc.

Life in Australia seemed to be going great for Mom and Kevin, but things began to change.

At first the changes were very small, like a joke about Kevin losing his car keys, a joke about Kevin getting old when not turning up for Sunday drinks after Saturday night drinks. Then I noticed that Kevin was getting sick quite often. Again nothing too alarming at the beginning, but these bouts of illness became more frequent and the diagnoses getting more obscure while one random virus followed the next.

As time went on, we could see a clear pattern evolving.....'Kevin is good and in great form.....Kevin is really sick.....Kevin is recovering.....Kevin is good and in great form'.

By year 5, Kevin could no longer work like he used to and seemed to be in hospital at least once a month. All the nurses in his 'new local' were getting to know him by his first name. It had become clear that the adventure was over and it was time for Kevin and Mom to return home.

As it turned out, I had planned a trip back home to Ireland and was leaving 10 days before they were due to leave and they would be gone when I returned. I had to say my goodbyes, wishing them all the best and a safe trip home as Kevin lay on his hospital bed and this time he had bird flu.

Again at this stage, none of us knew for certain what the future had in store for Kevin but quietly, I think we all knew that it wasn't going to be positive and life was never going to be as it was during those early years in Aus.

Since then, every phone call with Mom consists of an update on Kevin, latest specialist, latest nightmares, latest pill and potions. It really sounded like as though Kevin who was once the life of the party was losing his vivacious personality and had become quite introvert and isolated.

I met with Kevin in Ireland 2 years later and I saw a noticeable difference in his physical appearance. He had aged quite a bit and I had only one night out with him but to my surprise he made it back to Australia with Mom last year. When I met him at Sydney airport, sadly the Kevin I greeted was a changed man. It had been 9 years since I had first picked him up at Sydney airport but to my shock it looked like 25 years had passed. Mom and Kevin stayed with us for a couple of weeks and while we all had a wonderful time, Kevin's ill-health was uppermost on our minds. On any previous trip Kevin would be the first one up in the morning, out drinking coffee on the balcony or off to the beach to enjoy the Sydney sunrise regardless of any big nights' out but this time, on a good day he would get up around noon.

From what I have seen of this disease, it is slow and painful and not just for Kevin, but my Mom, his family, friends and anyone who knew Kevin, from when he was 'Kevin Quaid' and not 'Kevin who suffers from LBD'.

Who knows what the future holds but one thing I know for certain is….'enjoy each day while you can'.

Shane

Michelle O'Connell

Stepdaughter

Kevin has been my Stepdad for nearly 20 years now but I knew him a lot longer. He was hard working, full of the joys of life and always up for new adventures.

One of his many adventures was emigrating to Australia with my Mom. It was fantastic having our whole family there, all at the same time.

I started to see changes in Kevin while we were living down under in Sydney. He seemed to be having a big battle on his hands with his health and had lots of visits to hospital because of illness.

We could all clearly see that he was unable to work for as long or as hard as he had been. We were living in the beautiful city of Sydney, so of course we took every opportunity to take lots of family photos. These photos confirmed to me that Kevin's health was gradually getting worse as it was plain to see a deterioration when looking at the different photos but I still didn't understand what was wrong with him. Each time he was admitted to hospital, I wondered, what now? There was always a real and reliable explanation for each stay but when discharged I could see very little recovery, at least one that might bring him back to the active person he once was.

Mom and Kevin had to eventually move back to Ireland due to Kevin's poor health and of course this confirmed what I was already thinking….this is serious.

Since their return home 3 years ago, Kevin's health has got progressively worse. Some days I call and everything seems normal and I think he looks great and back to himself, but unfortunately there are the other days, too many to mention when he looks so sick and frail.

He can get very agitated and confused, therefore I never know what to expect on any given day, it really is 'One day at a time'. He can be very emotional at times but I know that he is in a lot of pain which breaks my heart. His natural vitality is slowly being drained away with this Lewy Body Dementia. My Mom, who

I'm sure Kevin will agree has been a huge support and thank God for her wonderful positivity which certainly keeps the show going.

I speak to Mom everyday but now when my phone rings, my first thought is….Is Kevin OK? Between trips to hospitals or doctors being called out of hours, or just a bad night of horrific nightmares, our conversations always come around to an update on Kevin.

I buried my head in the sand long enough but the reality was too raw for me to even think that Kevin may not know me or be around for as long as I just assumed he would be.

I love you dearly Kevin and pray for you and Mom every day and I feel really blessed to have you as my Stepdad.

Michelle O'Connell

Tom Quaid

Brother

My brother Kevin has LBD Lewy Body Dementia, I am living in Australia and Kevin is living in Ireland. We facetime each other every week or two and we have done this for a number of years, especially when Kevin lived in Sydney for a couple of years. When Kevin told me he was diagnosed, I got off the phone and thought, shit Kev has dementia, but people with dementia live for years and it's a slow boat to the end, but when my wife who is a nurse explained it to me, well my world really turned upside down. I also went online and My God this prognosis was incredible.

Kevin, my big brother all my life, someone that I looked up to as a young boy growing up, had this disease that is fast, aggressive and holds no boundaries. All the problems that come with it are just horrific. This disease is horrific for the person with it and the entire family and circle of friends associated with the sufferer.

Kevin was always the life and soul of the party a great man for the craic and always would give you the shirt of his back, even when he didn't have it.

Growing up we had our ups and downs like all families and all siblings but we never stopped trying and never stopped loving each other, he will always be my big brother. Kevin visited me in Perth last year and I thought that we were going to be able to go out, have a few beers and just have the craic (somewhat muted) like the good old days but poor Kev spent his time in beautiful Perth in bed for 3 days from the cocktail of prescribed drugs and a shit disease.

He got off the plane at the airport and my wife had told me to expect a huge change in Kevin and My God she was not wrong. My heart broke when I saw him as he had aged and looked so unwell. The following day we went for breakfast and I drove him around to show off my new business projects, but instead I listened to Kevin telling me how ill he was, how low he felt (suicidal), violent thoughts and horrific dreams, which just completely destroyed our time together. He told me about his plans for his death and decisions that he and his poor wife Helena had to discuss and make. I never thought that someone like Kevin could or would be in a position like this with all this terrible negativity in his life.

After spending the next 3 days and nights in bed being cared for by my lovely wife Julie, Kevin was just about able to fly to Sydney to his wife Helena and family. We managed to spend one evening with each other again on their return to Ireland and it was good but unfortunately not like the old days.

This disease is horrific and week by week I see a change in Kevin, and not a good change. I love my brother very much and I hope that there will be a cure found for this terrible disease in the near future, as people don't deserve this end to their life.

I hope Kevin gets to see his book completed and I hope people can get some relief or even a better understanding from his words and feelings.

I wish sufferers with LBD all the best and that you have a peaceful end when the time comes as I know your road has been a hard one

Tom Quaid

Michael Walsh

A true friend

It's difficult to put into words a friendship that started the first day we met, almost 25 years ago. On that day Kevin and I became brothers, there was just a bond that has grown over the years. The adventures and fun we have had over them years has given us laughs, tears and fabulous memories. When I think of our friendship I think of 2 Limerick lads in a family of Cork women.

I remember the holidays, adventures, jobs, businesses, cars, nights' out, occasions, weddings, births and unfortunately several funerals. Through all these events and years, Kevin's fun loving and impulsive personality is what I remember the most, of course his short fuse has given me many funny memories also!!

As the years have rolled by Kevin has had to face his biggest challenge with the diagnosis of Lewy Body Dementia. Unfortunately when I call to see my friend I am unsure as to which man I shall meet, the fun-loving adventurer or the man battling to keep his sanity. LBD has taken a firm grip of my auld pals' life and is affecting everyone connected to his life. It has stolen my friend and all the things we used to do like afternoons trying to play golf, nights' out in bars, family occasions, weekends away etc. Gone are the days of an impulsive trip or journey. Kevin can no longer drive and sometimes he isn't able for travelling, or the stairs, or the noise etc.

There are times he looks like his old self but just physically isn't able to go places, or even just get out of bed to have a coffee with me. At best he can chat and be alert but other times he can be illogical and angry. Kevin gets very emotional nowadays and more often than not tears seem to flow on many of our conversations. I fear for the future and the anger this illness has enraged in him, the depression, the lows it takes him to and I worry for him as the illness progresses.

I don't know where this journey is going to take him next or the many challenges Kevin still has to face but I will do my best to remain strong for him and keep reminding him of the good times.

Kevin is a loyal friend to me and I will not let him walk this journey alone and can only hope he never forgets how loved he is.

Mike

CHAPTER NINETEEN

Caregiving

Keep hope alive

&

Take care of the carer

When Kevin was first diagnosed, I knew very little about Lewy Body Dementia (LBD). Little did I know that this word would become my every waking thought within a few short years.

As Kevin's wife and carer, I can clearly see that this progressive degenerative neurological condition namely LBD, is not just one that leads to memory loss but is unpredictable, devastating and relentless. On a bad day or even in a bad moment, the situation may appear hopeless, but I have found that for me starting my day with a little meditation and some alone time to ground myself, sets me up for the day ahead and what living with a sufferer of LBD may bring.

The only way to deal with an LBD sufferer is to live one day at a time, accepting what the day or night might throw at me to the best of my ability and the best of my ability can be different on any given day. There are days when I grieve the personality change in Kevin and I grieve for the man that I met, fell in love with, married and have shared my life with for the past 18 years. In those times, I find myself barely holding on with my finger tips to the few positive thoughts that are left but I am determined to enjoy as much as LBD allows us to, in the time we have remaining.

My brother Paddy, who lives in San Francisco ends his phone calls saying 'Is e mar a ta se' which in English means 'it is what it is' I have used these words as my mantra to help me accept what is now my reality, caregiving.

Living as a carer to my husband with LBD 24/7 is like climbing a mountain. Some days when on a plateau the journey is pleasant but very often and very soon we re-emerge at another steep incline having to face yet another facet of this illness. Kevin is nervous at home alone and he is also nervous of the dark. This means I do not have the same social life I once had as it is dependent on how well he is that determines my ability to leave home, if only for a few hours. It is also important to acknowledge how tired I am and how often times because of this I avoid meeting others, hence making the life of a carer quite isolating.

LBD is an unpredictable foe and I never know what to expect on any given day or night. Not only is this disease unpredictable, but it also presents itself in many different ways. The presentation of this illness can vary not only from day to day but from moment to moment.

With LBD, some days Kevin is his old self but yet on other days he is unrecognisable both physically and emotionally. Due to this ever changing condition, I often feel like a fraud when telling family and friends how unwell he is, only to have them be met by the old Kevin when they come to visit the day after. In truth, there have been many times where I have even questioned my own sanity and asked myself 'did I imagine how bad he was'?

The symptoms of LBD are so varied that I have outlined what I see in Kevin in the following list:

Agitation, anxiety.

Blood pressure, blurred vision.

Confusion, changes in alertness, chest pain.

Depression, distress, delusion, delirium, dizziness, decline in abilities, drowsiness.

Emotional, excessive daytime sleepiness.

Frustration, false beliefs, frightened, fluctuating cognitive abilities.

Hearing problems, hot flushes.

Insomnia, impaired thinking, irritability, isolation.

Kidney infections.

Lack of concentration, lack of decision making abilities, lack of judgement, loss of enthusiasm, loss of balance.

Memory loss, mood changes.

Noise sensitivity, nervousness, night sweats.

Pain, personality change, physical changes.

Rem Sleep Behaviour Disorder (RBD)

At times this can be very frightening, especially when Kevin sees me as an intruder in our home while acting out his nightmares.

Reasoning problems, rigid muscles, rapidly changing symptoms, reduced attention span.

Shuffling walk, slowness of movement, slurred speech, sickness, sudden outbursts, suicidal, shaky handwriting.

Tremor, trouble initiating movement, trouble interpreting visual perceptions of space.

Unsteady gait, unpredictable nature, unresponsive, unable to drive, unable to do some tasks.

Viruses....Kevin has already outlined these in detail.

Visual hallucinations....in that moment, this is Kevin's reality.

Walking problems, wakefulness.

In conclusion, while no one can deny that caring for someone you love who suffers from LBD is hugely difficult, isolating and at times an overwhelming task, there is always hope. Hope comes when a memory resurfaces, a walk isn't too difficult, a photograph is recognised, a laugh can be shared and the man I married resurfaces to share a tender moment. To all of you reading this who may also be caring for your loved one, keep it in the day, know that your best is always good enough and always remember you are not alone.

celtichelena@y7mail.com

Addresses you may find useful

The Alzheimer Society of Ireland

1800 341 341

www.alzheimer.ie

The Crystal Project, Mallow, Co Cork

022 58700

www.crystalproject.ie

Carebright, Bruff, Co. Limerick

061 602 700

www.carebright.ie

Pieta House

1800 247 247

www.pieta.ie

Samaritans Ireland

116 123

www.samaritans.ie

Childhood Sexual Abuse

01 662 4070

www.oneinfour.ie

Printed in Great Britain
by Amazon

78913580R00119